To Sherree

One of the

## STILL HALF MY SIZE !!

Women I know !!

Enjoy the Ride

Big hugs
x Susie

First published in 2018 by New Holland Publishers
London • Sydney • Auckland

131–151 Great Titchfield Street, London WIW 5BB, United Kingdom
1/66 Gibbes Street, Chatswood, NSW, 2067, Australia
5/39 Woodside Ave, Northcote, Auckland, 0627, New Zealand

newhollandpublishers.com

A record of this book is held at the British Library and the National Library of
Australia.

ISBN 9781921024511

Group Managing Director: Fiona Schultz
Publisher: Alan Whiticker
Project Editor: Liz Hardy
Designer: Andrew Davies
Production Director: James Mills-Hicks
Cover photo: Chris Howley
Cover photo: Make-up and hair by Jacqueline Hutton, glindawand.com.au
Printer: Hang Tai Printing Company Limited

10 9 8 7 6 5 4 3 2 1

Keep up with New Holland Publishers on Facebook
facebook.com/NewHollandPublishers

# *Still* HALF MY SIZE

THE THINKING PERSON'S DIET

## SUSIE ELELMAN

NEW
HOLLAND

This book is dedicated to my late parents

Annemarie and Bill,

whose weaknesses I have inherited

and from whose strengths I constantly draw.

# CONTENTS

have always seen Susie Elelman as an angel with attitude. She's kind, generous, talented and a good friend. The other bonus is that she is honest and upfront. You know where you stand with Susie. I've stood with her on two television networks, Seven and Ten. She is one of the few people at home in both the news and commercial areas of television and radio.

It was a couple of years before I was aware that this beautiful woman is much more than a television talent. Her life story is fascinating. Now she shares it with us all.

If you're down and need to get up off the canvas, if life is starting to overtake you and it seems that dreams don't come true, be inspired by Susie Elelman. I am proud to call her a friend.

Enjoy her book and tell your friends! I'm sure that just like the Logie outfits that stop a nation, all will be revealed!

— Bert Newton

# INTRODUCTION

My first book *Half My Size: The Thinking Person's Diet* was published in 2005 and detailed how I'd shed in excess of 50 kilograms and kept it off for ten years.

Yes, I've lost more than Posh Spice weighs, which probably also equates to both the Olsen twins. Since then it's been an ongoing effort on my part to try and maintain my weight and remain half my size. I share my steps to success in this new book *Still Half My Size* and also the reasons behind the times when I didn't succeed.

More than once, in more recent times, I allowed myself to expand a few dress sizes, especially through winter, but never have I been twice my size again. Nevertheless, these failures still needed to be addressed and *Still Half My Size* examines the changes I've made, especially to my food fuel daily intake, that have made me half my size again and curbed the massive overeating and uncontrollable sugar cravings I've battled with for most of my life.

While the US is still leading the way as being the most obese nation on earth, it's alarming to learn that Australia is not too many percentage points behind with more than 60 per cent of all Aussie adults and more than a quarter of children obese or overweight.

But I've been partially to blame by being a big contributor to that growing statistic. For much of my life I was overweight and hating myself for it. That led me to try all sorts of weird and wonderful ways to get rid of that weight, with varying degrees of short-term success. More often than not I'd not only regain the weight but I'd generally add a few more kilos for extra measure. Now all that's changed and I'm thrilled to say that I'm STILL half my size.

My childhood battle with the bulge (I was size 14 at fourteen years of age) continued for long periods throughout my adult life and as you'll see from the photo gallery in this book, I've owned and worn every dress size from a 22 down to a 10–12.

In the early 1990s I was carrying in excess of 50 kilos more than I am now and this book describes the simple lifestyle changes that I have put in place to help reduce my size and change my shape.

Over the subsequent decades I've managed to maintain my weight for the most part but there have been times when my size has fluctuated enormously, when I've gone off the rails and back to my bad old eating habits. As soon as I start eating the right food fuel mix, along with regular exercise, I become the ever-shrinking woman again.

It would be impossible to hazard a guess as to the number of single column centimetres that magazines and newspapers have collectively dedicated to talking about weight loss and body image, not to mention the radio and television coverage. I've taken up quite a few of those column centimetres myself and copped a lot of media flack over my size. Some of those tough times are described in this book but I'm also a great believer in the old adage by Joseph P Kennedy and the message Jeff Fenech often writes on his boxing gloves when he signs them: 'When the going gets tough, the tough get going'.

This book is not designed to get you to live like me. Quite the contrary! You will actually have more of a chance of succeeding if you do it your way.

I'm hoping you'll learn to value your body and your mind like you would an expensive, prized possession – the analogy I use throughout this book is between a luxury car and our body. This book arms you with easy-to-use tools that allow you to carry out your ongoing commitment to reach and maintain your ideal size and shape.

I examine why some of us overeat and what triggers overeating for me. We analyse your food fuel and what mix is best to keep your motor running at peak performance. Included are simple steps that can be put in place so you don't have to deny yourself the things you enjoy. As well, I've suggested some interesting ways to burn off your fuel intake so you look and feel good about yourself on both the inside and the outside.

Does change push you out of your comfort zone and sometimes cause you uncomfortable emotions of fear and panic and the feeling of being out of control? These feelings can often trigger comfort and overeating behaviours to recur, which can result in us falling back into old habits. There's a focus in my book on willpower, self-esteem and positive thinking and tips on how to set goals and stay on track.

I've included lots of exciting twenty-first century scientific findings and discoveries that help explain so much more about weight management and why not all of it is within our control. But rest assured it can be.

You'll learn what foods can change the chemicals in our brain to make it extremely difficult, sometimes impossible, for us to summon the willpower needed to not overindulge, and in turn, to not shed the kilos nor keep them off.

My research has uncovered how the Big Food companies specifically employ food scientists and spend bucket loads of money double blind testing 'human guinea pigs' with various amounts of fat, sugar and salt to find what's commonly referred to in the food industry as the 'bliss point' in their food. The 'bliss point' is reached when the right combination of these foods and flavours makes us crave it more and more, rather than it satisfying us. Potentially these manufactured foods are as addictive as hard drugs and cigarettes and extremely harmful to our long-term health as well.

*Still Half My Size* isn't just a look through my rear-vision mirror, sharing my stories with you; all the interviews with high-profile celebrities, who generously gave their time and expertise in *Half My Size*, have been included in *Still Half My Size*.

These extremely talented and experienced contributors include: champion marathon swimmer Shelley Taylor-Smith, best-selling author Tara Moss, Elle Macpherson's mum Fran Macpherson, Channel Ten newsreader Sandra Sully, *Studio 10* host Jessica Rowe, world-champion boxer Jeff Fenech, extraordinary athlete and motivational speaker John Maclean, former rugby-league star Wayne Pearce, ironman Trevor Hendy, and breakfast radio hosts, Dave Gorr and the late Phebe Irwin, who highlight their shiftworking experiences and the devastating effects it had on their weight and overall health. You'll find celebrity tips at the end of each chapter and their full interviews in Chapter 9 'Secrets from the stars'.

There are some additional interviews I was excited to conduct specifically for this book.

Pete Evans the award-winning internationally renowned chef, restaurateur, published author, television presenter and judge on Channel 7's *My Kitchen Rules,* who's often nicknamed Paleo Pete (and I believe unnecessarily maligned by many), shares his passion and beliefs that food is medicine in Chapter 3 'We are what we eat'.

The thought-provoking interviews I've had recently on talkback radio with Tasmanian orthopaedic surgeon and founder of nofructose.com Dr Gary Fettke, have had the most profound impact on me making the vital changes needed to my daily food fuel mix to finally stop the cravings, overeating and never feeling full.

Going through menopause singlehandedly caused me to go off-road big time, it was one of the hardest journeys for me to take in so many ways. In Chapter 7 I detail my out-of-control eating and weight gain and the depressing changes to my body shape and size that I endured alongside the night sweats, hot flushes and all my other hideous menopause symptoms.

Another Gary impressed me immensely; Dr Gary Aaron from the Australian Menopause Centre (AMC), who is all about anti-ageing in the most natural way. Dr Gary explains simply and easily what happens to women in the lead up, during and after menopause and why it has such an adverse impact on our weight and body shape in Chapter 7 'Managing the menopause madness'.

No matter what size we are right now, many of us want to look like we're even slimmer. The incredibly talented international dress designer Christopher Essex, who made my original jaw-dropping Logie outfits, sadly passed away in 2006, but not before he shared lots of his simple, timeless styling and fashion tips to help us look slimmer and stylish. Christopher's dressing to suit your size and shape tips will help create the illusion you are trimmer – without even having to shed a kilogram! You'll find Christopher Essex's styling tips along with celebrity photographer Belinda Rolland's 'tricks of the trade' showing what poses make us look our slimmest in photos in Chapter 10 'Smoke & mirrors'.

You might even want to head straight to the unsealed section, Chapter 11 'Add SEX and double your results', to see how many kilograms you do burn and how sex stacks up to other activities. It's filled with helpful tips from Dr Rosie King, who emphasises the important role sex can play in weight loss and fitness and how it can also improve your self-esteem, body image, and your moods. This in turn can help with weight loss and fitness.

Do you like what you see when you look in the mirror? If the answer's no then you're not alone. I used to think like that but not anymore. This book details simple changes that I've discovered that can be easily implemented and incorporated into your life to immediately improve the way you look and feel. The aim of this book is not to tell you how to do anything … but rather to show you ways that you can realistically achieve results, your way!

Good luck.

– Susie

# CHAPTER 1

# CONFESSIONS OF A FOODAHOLIC

I f I cast my mind back as far as I can remember, I was always referred to as either fat or plump or, heaven forbid, pleasantly plump. In fact it was those last two words delivered by my family doctor when I was a teenager that first prompted me to embark on my roller-coaster ride of consciously losing weight.

I use the roller-coaster analogy because I'm really not keen on them at all; actually, to say that I'm terrified of them would be an understatement. I'm scared of heights so going up a three-rung ladder to change a light bulb used to always be a challenge. But today I think I'd rather take on the biggest ride in any amusement park than go on another roller-coaster ride with my weight.

The wear and tear on my body after constantly changing weight is bad enough but it's the psychological damage that I've put myself through that I believe is even more detrimental to my health. One of my closest friends said to me only recently, 'You've lost and gained weight so many times you could have had five or six children.'

I've lost count of the number of rumours that used to go around about me being pregnant each time I did gain weight, but as I don't have any children of my own, I can't blame them, just me.

As successful as I have been at eventually losing the weight, I would only manage to maintain it for what seemed like a very short time and then, invariably, it would creep back on and before I knew it I'd gained even more weight than I'd just lost. If I were to stereotype myself, I guess you could call me a foodaholic.

## By my own admission 'I am an addict'

I can remember the first time I stood up and said those words in public; I was more nervous than the first time I gave a public speech. When I first admitted publicly I was an addict, I was in my thirties and it was in a meeting room at the back of a church hall with a group of about 25 people, each of whom introduced themselves only by their first name and who shared one thing in common with me: they were all addicts too. Despite my many years of experience in public speaking, in that church hall meeting room my mouth was dry, my palms were very sweaty, my heart was beating extra fast and I certainly couldn't make eye contact with anyone. When the words came out of my mouth it was like someone else was speaking. Was this really me speaking, and was this the real me speaking? When I sat down I had the strangest emotional experience; tears just streamed down my face. They were not tears of pain or tears of sadness, they were tears of relief.

It's easier to disclose a secret to strangers than to friends and family. I'd heard the expression 'a weight being lifted off your shoulders' many times but I think that was one of the times in my life that I can actually recall feeling that very sensation. I left that meeting mentally and physically exhausted. It felt like I'd been run over by a steamroller but I also sensed a lightness in my heart and a feeling of hope. While I knew I'd feel better in the long run for going there, I can only describe the experience as an uncomfortable comfort. It was clear from everyone who shared their stories during the meeting that they had their own impairment – some great, some small.

One of my big downfalls in the past, although I never recognised it as a downfall then, was to put too much focus on others, sometimes at my own expense. I believe most women, and especially mothers, instinctively put others ahead of themselves and I'm now aware that I can channel far too much energy towards others and not enough on myself.

It was easy to do that at the meeting, with all the lovely, welcoming people that I had met. That's why I had to be very careful not to lose focus on what I wanted and needed to achieve. It's taken me many, many years, filled with lots of different life experiences and counselling since that first meeting, to be able to finally admit publicly that I'm an addict.

Now, for the first time in my life, I've accepted what I've done in the past and I don't care what people think of me, or how they judge me, as long as I like me then I'm doing just fine.

I'm writing this book to share my experiences in the hope that it may help others to overcome their own addictions. Accepting yourself, I believe, is the most important breakthrough you can make mentally in order to stay on the 'straight and narrow'.

This quote, credited to the 18th century German philosopher GWF Hegel, reinforces that message to me: 'Thus to be independent of public opinion is the first formal condition of achieving anything great.'

Please don't get me wrong, I value people's opinions and I take their advice on board and am constantly learning. But at the end of the day, when push comes to shove, there is only one person's opinion I ultimately care about, listen to and act upon and that's my own.

Accepting myself has been a real shift in paradigm for me because I've had to believe in my inner self and trust my judgments and instincts, which in the past I've so often suppressed, questioned or doubted.

Being an addict can be a very isolating and depressing experience. Aside from the shame, the guilt and the feeling of being a failure that often overwhelms you, there's also the tendency to get very sneaky in order to hide your problem from the people around you. Others try not to judge, but they can't always help it; and despite the fact that your closest friends and family love you dearly, they can often make matters worse when, consciously or unconsciously, they leave you with feelings of guilt as a result of their efforts to support or help you.

When trying to fight an overwhelming desire that has an unadmitted stranglehold on your life, I have found these emotional pressures may serve to reinforce the need to conceal addictive behaviours and increase the feelings of failure and being different and irresponsible.

Emotional pressures and low self-esteem or self-worth often trigger addictive disorders, which then may be unintentionally fuelled and perpetuated by well-meaning family and friends. That's why organisations like Alcoholics Anonymous, Narcotics Anonymous, Gamblers Anonymous and Overeaters Anonymous all have support groups and counselling for the addict, as well as for families and loved ones.

Of all addictions a food addiction is, without a doubt, the one that is the hardest to camouflage and to keep under control.

## Why do only some people get addicted and not others?

I'd become very rich if only I had the answer to that question, but I do believe an addiction is a complex illness that starts in our genes but is not just that in isolation. Along with this genetic predisposition there's a physical, psychological and/or emotional trigger that causes sustained elevated stress levels and an ever lowering of self-esteem. That, combined with a conscious or unconscious belief that this trigger cannot be overcome, leads a pre-addict to focus on a short-term, 'feel-good' behaviour, which, over time, becomes more frequent and more regular, and is needed in ever-increasing doses. Before you know it, a dependency develops.

It's been my observation that most addicts have more than one addiction. Many drug addicts smoke cigarettes.

Compulsive gamblers and alcoholics can easily combine their addictions at the one licensed venue. Let's not forget the other uncontrollable urges, which are often not treated as seriously as drug or alcohol addictions, such as eating disorders, over-exercising and uncontrollable shopping. One major problem that I discovered in trying to control my addictions is that unconsciously I am looking for short-term fixes and not tackling the underlying problem; you can end up swapping one addiction for another.

It was Becky Lu Jackson's book *Dieting – A Dry Drunk* that showed me how my eating disorder was the most difficult addiction to control. Becky Lu explains that for an alcoholic it is sobriety, a drug addict strives to be clean, but a foodaholic can't abstain from eating food altogether or we'll die.

We are confronted and challenged by our addiction each time we come in contact with food. In my case that's at least three to five times a day when I feel the pangs of hunger, not to mention the number of times when I've drawn on food for comfort or enjoyment, irrespective of whether I was hungry or not. My abstinence has had to be twofold; firstly, to initially totally abstain from the foods that I can't control (and that's a pretty big list as you'll see in Chapter 3 'We are what we eat'), as well as more generally abstaining from overeating.

## So when did my 'foodiction' begin?

Long before I can even remember – and that is a long time!

I was already doomed by centuries of inherent social behaviour. Anyone from a European family, like me, will know that the first thing you do when the doorbell rings is think, what have I got in the fridge or the cupboard to offer my visitors?

Our family was far from rich yet there was always plenty of food on the table. I found that our family activities at home were mostly focused around the dining table or kitchen bench and food, yummy fattening food, was a huge and natural part of this. Everything was in bowls in the centre of the table and we helped ourselves, which meant no-one monitored the quantity of food I ate or how many times I went back for seconds and thirds, including me. In fact, we were encouraged to eat up, and if you were well-rounded, all the better. No wonder eating is still one of my favourite pastimes!

I've always enjoyed food and the more exotic the better. I was exposed to an enormous variety of tastes while I was growing up and have been able to expand both my palate and my waistline through many decades of international travel. I'm hoping for many more overseas adventures in the future but I'll do them a little differently and make sure the only excess baggage I bring home will be my luggage.

## Feeling like a fish out of water

In the early years I sort of lived two lives; one, inside our home with all the European culture, food, strict rules and customs that my parents were raised on and passed onto us. The other was when I stepped out of our front door and desperately tried to blend in and be as Anglo-Saxon as most of my other Australian friends. That's one area where I had open conflict with my father. I guess while it was relatively easy to take Mum and Dad out of Europe, it wasn't quite so easy to take Europe out of Mum and Dad.

Dad was born in Warsaw in 1922, a Polish Jew, who as a teenager witnessed most of his family, including his mother, being murdered by the Nazis. Dad was a holocaust survivor who carried severe physical and mental scars from his years in concentration camps in Germany and Poland including Auschwitz. When they arrived in Australia as refugees Dad could speak eleven languages, four fluently, it's just a shame not one of them was English.

Mum was more like the United Nations and not just because she always tried to keep the peace at home and constantly stuck up for us kids, but also because she's very multinational. Born in Herten on the German–Polish border in 1924, at age four Mum moved to Ulm on the Danube near Bavaria after her Polish-Jewish father died. Mum was raised a Catholic mainly by her aunt and sometimes by her French mother and German stepfather. Mum could speak German, French, Polish and very little schoolgirl English.

Mum and Dad met at the end of the war in Germany. By the late 1940s they decided to leave Europe and start a new life far away from the horror and the aftermath of the war and they qualified to go to either America or Australia.

Neither of them knew much about Australia, nor were there any tourist bureaus to get brochures. It wasn't until decades later that the successful Hoges 'put a shrimp on the barbie' campaign started and Oprah and Ellen weren't even born then.

So Dad looked at a map of the world and chose Australia primarily for its geographical location. I think our former Prime Minister Paul Keating put it most eloquently when he described us as 'the arse end of the world'.

With a two-year-old in hand, a suitcase filled with clothes, and whatever belongings would fit into a small trunk, Mum and Dad took a train from Germany to Italy, where my eldest brother Leon contracted chicken pox. They were quarantined and had to use up their limited savings to survive until they were cleared to board a converted American tanker called the *General Blatchford* for six weeks on the high seas to come to Australia.

When they arrived at Circular Quay they had the sum total of five pounds (the equivalent of about $10) in their pockets. Mum didn't have much time to recover from her motion sickness because as soon as they were processed, they were immediately transferred by train to a camp in Bathurst. Both Mum and Dad had grown up in big, cosmopolitan cities and Mum had travelled extensively with her aunt throughout Europe as a child, but nothing could have prepared them for the enormous culture shock of Australia. They realised they had a whole lot of adjusting to do.

Dad only lasted one day in the camp at Bathurst before heading back to Sydney where he found accommodation and work and they settled at Mona Vale on Sydney's northern beaches. Three years later Mum fell pregnant again and Eddie was born in 1953. But after four boys (sadly two of my brothers passed away in Germany) Mum was desperate for a girl so she kept trying and, against all odds, I followed fifteen months later. Apparently I was no lightweight, weighing almost nine pounds, and Mum told me I didn't give her an easy time at birth either.

It was tough for my parents to raise three children, in a foreign country, without any support or extended family to call on, but they learnt English as quickly as they could because Mum and Dad knew that was one of the vital keys to assimilating. They were keen to be 'Aussies', and not only became naturalised Australians as soon as they could, but they both also made very valuable contributions to their local community. However we still lived like Europeans at home, especially when it came to food.

In the early years, long before there were any supermarkets and before delicatessens were in just about every suburb, Dad would regularly travel, firstly by a series of buses and then years later by car, from Mona Vale to Bondi to go to the European delicatessens to get foods they were familiar with, like wursts, salami, herrings, smoked eel, black bread and Dad's favourite, goose fat.

To say my dad was strict would be an understatement and I grew up being terrified of him. One thing Dad made us do when we were very young was to eat everything that was on our plate whether we liked it or not, or whether we were full or not. And believe me, he made you sit there until you finished it, no matter how long it took and there certainly wasn't any dessert for my delay. I understand that Dad was doing what he thought was right and what he'd obviously been taught.

Most of my childhood friends, like me, had a sweet tooth and many of their parents would also successfully get them to eat a healthy meal by rewarding them with dessert only when that was finished.

Growing up, most Aussie kids copped the 'think about all the starving children in Africa' routine, to make them eat and not waste our food. Instead, we were made well aware of the years that Dad starved in concentration camps and Mum lived on food rations. Also, Dad didn't want us to be fussy eaters and my parents definitely didn't have any spare time or money to waste on different foods to suit everyone's taste. While I can appreciate all that, I also believe it taught me more bad behaviours than good ones, including overeating and delayed gratification. I learnt to eat the things I didn't like, or liked least, first, then save the best bits until last in order to push through feeling full and finish what was on my plate.

Eating fast was another way I found I could fit it all in, and I still eat my food too quickly today. Sometimes I go into overdrive and I just shovel it down and don't even realise what I'm doing. I've often read that you should put your knife and fork down between each mouthful and that it takes your stomach about twenty minutes to tell your brain that it's full. When I'm at home I use smaller plates and bowls to reduce my portion sizes and smaller knives, forks and spoons, and sometimes even chopsticks, to slow down the eating process, and it works.

My parents had very strong accents and broken English. As they had just arrived from Germany with our German-sounding last name ending in 'man', we were falsely branded Nazis or Nazi sympathisers. Despite the atrocities Dad had to endure at the hands of the Nazis and Mum being buried alive and unconscious for three months (yes she was it is an amazing story) when American bombs hit her home town in Germany during World War II, both Mum and Dad were still being vilified right here in Australia.

Children can be so cruel and with the help of my mother's mantra of 'sticks and stones may break my bones but names will never hurt me', I'd try to ignore the chanting of horrible and hurtful names. In those post war years, racial prejudice was prevalent and I experienced my fair share of verbal and physical taunts as a 'fat wog' kid growing up in the ritzy northern beaches of Sydney during the late fifties, sixties and early seventies.

I always knew I looked a bit different from other non-Indigenous Aussie with my jet-black hair and olive skin, but I also knew I was born in Manly hospital, which is why from a very young age I was confused as to why these bullies would keep insisting that I go back to where I came from.

Mum and I would spend many hours together while I was growing up discussing various subjects, and prejudice was often one of them. I still can't understand how anyone can be judged on the colour of their skin or their sexuality. You have about as much chance of changing those as you do your eye colour yet other people take issue with them.

Even though I was a year younger than most of my classmates, you would never know by my size.

Eddie and I were often asked if we were twins and despite him being fifteen months older than me people always believed him when he said I was older. Being bigger never concerned me when I was young because Mum was the most talented dressmaker and designer. We loved to window shop or go through her favourite *Burda* German fashion magazines, which were always a season ahead, and she'd come back home and make me everything that was fashionable; they would fit my shape perfectly, helping conceal the extra kilos.

What it was really hiding was a scared fat little wog kid, who was using food as a barrier to combat being bullied, victmised and beaten up. I've continued that same default pattern of comfort eating whenever I've had to deal with most major crises in my adult life.

> 'No-one can make you feel inferior without your consent.'
> — ELEANOR ROOSEVELT

I now realise that throughout my life at times I've allowed people's judgments about me to affect my behaviours and decisions. Having yo-yoed so many times with my weight it was hard not to convince myself that I was going to be anything other than fat and no matter how hard I tried, there was nothing I could do about it long term. I've spent most of my life either on a diet or going off a diet and I'm sure I'm not alone in describing some of the psychological games we put ourselves through in order to lose weight.

When I was off my diet I'd favour either the 'Pasta Diet' – any time I'd walk past a cake shop I'd have to go in, or the 'Seafood Diet' – see food and I'd eat it. I'd often joke that I only ate 'one meal a day' – it started in the morning and ended at night.

When I was 'on a diet' I'd put myself through torture eating the most ridiculous combinations. There have been some diet doozeys. Take the grapefruit diet, for example. It wouldn't be the right season and I'd never seem to be able to choose the sweet, juicy grapefruits. Instead, every mouthful seemed to suck all the saliva out of my mouth and replace it with a bitter aftertaste. I'm not surprised that one didn't last long!

But without a doubt, for me the worst would have to be the Israeli army diet, which required you to eat nothing but apples for the first two days and, if my memory serves me correctly, they were even supposed to be the same variety, then two days of nothing but cheese, followed by two days of nothing but chicken. I'm not totally sure what the final two days were, I think it was lettuce but I never got that far. I wonder if anyone ever did?!

In my early teens, when I set out on my first diet, which I realise now is the worst thing you can do, there wasn't a lot of information around and certainly not a lot of healthy alternatives on the market. I can remember paying a fortune for these dreadful tasteless rolls that I could barely bite into that were supposed to be help with weight loss. They didn't work for me; all they achieved was to make me feel miserable and hungrier.

Sadly, I even used laxatives that you could buy in the supermarket. All they'd given me was a bad case of the runs and I didn't manage to lose an ounce on them.

Throughout the course of my weight loss roller-coaster ride, I've tried every diet pill on the market and had varying degrees of success but nothing ever seemed to work for me long term.

> 'If at first you don't succeed you are running about average.'
> - M H ANDERSON

## Binge eating

For me, there are moments when all sensible and rational thinking about food goes out the window to be replaced by an overwhelming and sometimes uncontrollable desire to consume as much high-fat or high-sugar food as possible, regardless of the long- and short-term detrimental effects it will have on me.

I've often wondered what causes binge eating and set out to try to find out what triggered these bouts and why they could override the hormonal signals we normally receive to regulate our appetite.

According to information I read in the *New England Journal of Medicine,* it would appear that binge eating could be in the genes. A study showed a link between a defective gene known as the melanocortin four receptor gene and overeating and morbid obesity. If you would like to read more, the full article is available from www.nejm.org (Volume 348:1160–1163 published 20 March 2003).

Learning this not only made interesting reading but has actually been a great comfort for me. It's scientific proof that I'm not to blame. Having substantiated evidence that my binge eating can be linked to genetics, or Mother Nature, or God as we understand him/her, means that I can now recognise and accept why it's happening and that it is out of my control and I need to put steps in place to overcome the triggers.

I've often half-jokingly said, 'I'd be thin if I could have chosen my parents' and, as the medical journal article indicates, there is evidence of the relationship between obesity and genetics. Now I'm living proof that you can overcome genetics to lose half your size and keep it off just by thinking a little differently.

## Comfort eating

Stress is one of the biggest triggers for my binge eating. Is it cosmic that stressed spelt backwards is desserts? And what's worse is I put weight on really quickly, in fact I've never had any trouble in that department.

In 1993 I easily gained 10 kilograms in just two weeks when my dad was dying. For two years before Dad's premature death he refused to speak to me over a silly remark I'd made at a Christmas lunch and if ever there was a time when I used food to comfort me, it was then. It was only five weeks before Dad's untimely death at the hand of a doctor that we started talking again. I continued to use food as a crutch in the two years that followed while I spent a great deal of that time communicating back and forth with the Professional Standards Committee of the Health Department. Four months before Mum passed away in August 1995 I was successful in having the doctor found guilty of medical negligence and the law changed, so no-one else will ever have to suffer the same horrendous death as my dad.

I can assure you Dad's death wasn't the first time I'd used food to comfort me and certainly was not the last. Often after a visit to my parents' place I'd call into the nearest service station for petrol and stock up on junk food that I would binge on as I made my way home. Tim Tams and Kettle chips were always my favourite. There are eleven Tim Tams in a regular packet (and nine in the fancy flavours) and I'd eat them all in one car-trip home and then dispose of the packaging, which made me somehow think that I could justify to myself that it didn't count.

I'm not proud to admit it but I've eaten three packets of Tim Tams in one sitting. And so as not to add insult to injury, I'd always wash it down with diet coke. Of course the only person I was kidding was me.

On the subject of diet soft drinks, you might think they're a better alternative to regular soft drinks laden with sugar but research out of the French National Institute of Health and Medical Research (INSERM) published in the *American Journal of Clinical Nutrition* suggests switching to artificially-sweetened drinks may not necessarily reduce your diabetes risk – in fact, it might make it worse. This new evidence comes from a study of more than 66,000 French women, who were all middle-aged or older when the research began and then had their health monitored over fourteen years. When the researchers compared women who drank diet soft drink with women who drank the same amount of regular soft drink, they found the risk of developing diabetes was higher for those who chose diet soft drinks.

There's evidence artificial sweeteners might trigger cravings for more sweet food resulting in weight gain too. These ideas were supported by a study in 2010 which showed that aspartame, the most common artificial sweetener in diet soft drinks, could trigger insulin peaks in the body similar to those triggered by sugar.

Research from the France study has shown users of artificial sweeteners have higher blood sugar levels on average than non-users but another sugar replacement, stevia, has been shown not to cause raised blood sugar or insulin levels.

Over the years my emotions, my hormones, my menstrual cycle, the full moon, stress and men are just some of the things that have impacted on my weight. I seem to be able to gain weight in a matter of microseconds, yet I know every second of every minute of every day of every month that I'm trying to get it off again.

People do constantly congratulate me on my achievement, but I also see it the other way around – as a reminder of the excess weight that I carried. What I'm most proud of is that while I've gained and lost a few dress sizes over the years since shedding over 50 kilograms, I haven't put it all back on again and more, like I have in the past. For the first time in my life I've finally found a more realistic view of the foods that trigger all my old bad habits.

Now if my weight fluctuates slightly – as it does for most people, especially women over the course of a month and even more so between summer and winter – I am able to take control and remain the size and shape I want to be.

I knew something would have to change for my weight to stay down and under my control. What I didn't know was that the biggest change had to be in my head and not my stomach; I had to change the way I thought.

A man who has sent me on many of my journeys of discovery is my brilliant general practitioner (GP) Dr Jim Turner. Dr Jim's the most wonderful compassionate man and such a well-respected practitioner, who has opened my eyes and my mind to the ways that I could change.

One of the things I finally realised was that I couldn't keep reacting like I did when I was a child, taking comfort in overindulging and not dealing with any difficult issue that was confronting me. Instead of hiding behind a family-sized block of chocolate, I had to make my inner child grow up and deal with these emotions like the external adult that I saw in the mirror or I was never going to be able to make any progress.

I also believe you can change inherent behaviour with cognitive therapy and NLP (Neuro Linguistic Programming) guru Laureli Blyth shares in more detail how you can teach yourself new skills in Chapter 5 'How do I say NO and mean it?'.

Today I make most of my stressful or difficult decisions by mentally taking myself up to sit on the moon and look down on the Earth, to try to view my problems more broadly and with a little detachment. You'll be amazed at the different perspective you can achieve when looking down from up there. I always try and look at it from the outside in. The spectators always see the game far better than the players do.

Maybe there is something you can identify with or relate to in this book. Perhaps reading it will make you confront issues of your own that you never even thought were linked to your weight, but please take comfort in the knowledge that as you take your own journey there is a 'light at the end of the tunnel'.

My obesity tunnel has been long, and for years my light looked like a pinhead spot far away in the distance. What I do know is that the darkness of the tunnel is behind me and I'm now standing in bright daylight – and that's how I intend to keep it.

What a shame I can't just rest on my laurels. Instead I've had to make an ongoing commitment, both mentally and physically, to remain the size and shape I desire, and I treat it like any other addiction and take it one day at a time.

# CHAPTER 2

# A FORK IN THE ROAD

'The real voyage of discovery consists not in seeking new landscapes, but in having new eyes.'

- MARCEL PROUST

The difference between successfully shedding 50 plus kilograms, which I documented in *Half My Size*, and all the other times that I've gained and lost and regained weight is that I've finally made some simple but significant decisions outside of the food I eat that have given me a much better mental approach to my weight management. In the past I've always thought I had good intentions, but really only gave it lip-service and it's always ended up the same way: with broken promises and disappointment and more weight gained than lost.

## Don't weigh yourself

One of the important changes I made was to throw away my scales and promise never to weigh myself again. Sounds a bit harsh? Well I needed to be. When I sat down to identify the things that triggered my emotions in relation to food, I realised that weighing myself was one of them.

It had become this tortuous ritual; every morning I would wake up, pee and then weigh myself, because I knew that was when I would weigh the least (unless I was feeling good about myself and then I might weigh myself much more often). That morning weigh-in then set the emotional agenda for the rest of the day and, depending on the results, I would either feel good or bad about myself.

Doing this every day meant that the fluctuation of weight loss or gain wasn't large but it became paramount and fuelled my ongoing mind-set about my weight. Having the scales was triggering my compulsion to weigh myself and then, by weighing myself, I was constantly making myself aware of how much I weighed. It was an unhealthy vicious cycle.

I even bought myself a set of talking scales once. I knew I was in real trouble when I got on them one day the voice said, 'One at a time please'.

All jokes aside, I did have talking scales and also bought Dad a set for Christmas one year in the early 1980s. Dad loved gadgets, another thing I inherited from him, and like most of my family he was obsessed with his weight.

My brother Eddie is the only one in the family who can eat anything and never gain weight. He's had the same size waist or smaller since high school. I used to ask Mum how that could have happened and why it couldn't have been me instead. Mum said that she did two things differently when she was pregnant with Eddie.

The first was to have her weight monitored. It was Mum's first pregnancy in Australia and our wonderful next-door neighbour Betty advised her to go to the local baby health clinic. Mum did this regularly throughout her pregnancy with Eddie. Mum had never worried about her weight during her first three pregnancies and the nurses encouraged and helped Mum keep her weight down during this one. Then when she fell pregnant with me she didn't feel the need to go back to the baby health centre, nor did she keep a close eye on her weight.

I was interested to read an article in *The Sunday Telegraph* newspaper (11 July 2004), which confirmed what Mum and I had often speculated: that there was a link between a mother's obesity during pregnancy and her child's risk of obesity. The article outlines a study by the University of Cincinnati that found the period before a mother conceives, the time during her pregnancy and the early stages of a child's life can all be crucial in preventing childhood obesity.

This was backed up in 2009 by the results of a further study conducted by the University of Queensland that found a link between excess weight gain by during pregnancy and a higher body mass index (BMI) reading in their children at 21 years of age.

The other thing Mum did differently during her pregnancy with Eddie was that she craved and ate massive amounts of raw oats. I'm not sure if the two are directly related but he was born with two front teeth. Mum suffered through all the agony and bruising to bravely keep on breastfeeding him.

Back to the talking scales, which were a big hit that Christmas. You could program in your weight and each time you selected your button and hopped on the scales, it would announce how much you weighed and then how much you had gained or lost. You could then program it to say either 'Have a nice day' (no prizes for guessing that they came from America) or 'goodbye'.

I decided to play a practical joke on Dad, as I knew he'd stand on them in front of us all as soon as he opened his present, so before I wrapped them I stood on them and recorded my weight under what would be his number. As I thought, Dad found a level spot in the centre of the room, hit the button I instructed him to and a robotic-sounding male voice with a slight American twang asked him to 'Please step on the scales'. After lots of laughter he managed to balance himself, as instructed ,and the same voice announced, 'Your weight is 123 kilograms, you have gained 36 kilograms, and have a nice day'.

Well the look on his face was a Kodak moment, and the hysterical laughter that followed more than justified the exorbitant amount of money I'd paid for them. It gave us all great amusement that Christmas Eve with each of us taking turns to have a go.

As much fun as we had with the scales around the Christmas tree that year, I didn't realise what a crutch these scales had become; and not a crutch to help me recover either but rather one that was hindering me.

Thinking about it, there wasn't a time in my life that I didn't have bathroom scales. Each time I'd walk into the bathroom, day or night, it would be the first thing that always caught my attention. Like a beacon that had some sort of force field, it would draw me closer and, before I knew it, I had taken that regrettable half-step onto the scales and was standing as still as I could, eyes fixed at the glass dome waiting patiently for that needle to stop rocking back and forth.

I'd even move the scales to a flatter spot hoping it was the flooring and not me that was the reason I was heavier than before. And I think that force field is around every set of scales because when I used the bathroom at friends' places I'd always be drawn to try their scales, mainly, I think, in the hope that mine might be wrong.

Throughout my weight loss roller-coaster ride, I've picked up a lot of information that has helped formulated my views, so it's not just my ongoing weight paranoia that stops me weighing myself.

How many times have you heard people say, 'Fat weighs more than muscle'? It's wrong of course.

A kilo of muscle tissue is the same weight as a kilo of fat, however, the difference is that muscle is more compact and takes up less room. Also, your weight is never the same over a seven-day cycle. Therefore, if you base your success or failure solely on what the scales say daily then you are fighting a never-ending battle that can't be won.

'Wow! Look at you! How much weight have you lost?' That's often the first comment people make to me, particularly if they haven't seen me off-camera before or they know me but haven't seen me for a while. To be honest I can't ever give an accurate answer, as I haven't weighed myself since 1995.

The heaviest weight I've ever recorded was more than 120 kilograms and I know I put on lots more kilos after that but wasn't game to find out how many more; I'm sure it would have been another 10 kilos at my heaviest.

I do know I've shed in excess of 50 kilograms, but I wouldn't know exactly how much and I'm thrilled to say I really don't care anymore. It's that shift in paradigm – no longer being obsessed with weighing myself – that has definitely helped me with my long-term recovery and ongoing weight management.

When I trained with Jeff Fenech at his gym, which I did just about every morning for more than five years, I'd see his boxers constantly getting on the scales, but they have a legitimate reason to do so. They have to make their weight division to fight. I don't and it's likely you don't either. Sometimes after training the boxers would suggest that I jump on the scales too but I never did as I didn't want to start that vicious cycle again. I no longer have that urge or need to know how much I weigh.

There are of course occasions when you do need to be weighed by others, generally by health professionals, or if you are going to a weight-loss centre or seeing a dietitian. I have no dramas with that. My GP Dr Jim always takes my blood pressure and puts me on his scales as a matter of course whenever I'm in his doctor's surgery.

When it happens to me, I choose not to look at the dial or ask how much I weigh. For instance, when I was weighed during the few times I've been lucky enough to spend an enlightening week or weekend at the Golden Door Health Retreat, I've turned around the other way and asked the personal trainers to simple record my weight on their documents and not on mine.

## Let your clothes be the judge

The easiest and best way to judge your size and shape is with your clothes. Even though the weight gain happens all over your body, I notice my clothes getting tight firstly around my waistline, hips and upper thighs.

While I was on the roller-coaster, if I felt my clothes getting tighter, I wouldn't examine what was causing it and then put positive changes in place to loosen them again. Instead, I'd take the easy option and go into my expansive wardrobe of clothes that varies in sizes to cope with the smaller me, the bigger me and everything in between.

Clothes are a great yardstick and often it's that special pair of jeans or little black dress that we love and want to get back into that is our benchmark for success, and it is always important to have a goal to work towards.

Often, however, we have unrealistic expectations of ourselves and others. I have a friend who used to drag out her wedding dress leading up to every wedding anniversary and then beat herself up if she couldn't fit into it. She had been married for almost twenty years with two children when she finally stopped trying to look the same as she did on her wedding day. To make matters worse her husband would always 'jokingly' hassle her about it. I know he loves her and probably meant well but seeing her reaction made me feel that his behaviour contributed to her insecurities.

## Only measure your waistline.

The best way to keep a track record of how you are progressing with your weight management is to simply take your waist circumference regularly, measuring at your navel.

Abdominal fat, or visceral fat that sits around your waist, is what medical experts all say is the most dangerous fat for us to carry as it surrounds all our internal organs and is associated with many serious health problems including cardiovascular disease, type 2 diabetes and increased blood pressure.

It's important that your waist measurement stays under 88 centimetres for women and 102 centimetres for men.

## At my heaviest!

The biggest size in clothing I've ever bought for myself was size 22. The one I remember the most was a skirt and jacket in a loud blue and white print and I can recall being delighted that the elasticised waistband was too big and had to be pinned in. It had a huge jacket with big padded shoulders and it hung over my huge frame, dwarfing all my trouble spots. By that stage, I'd lost sight of the fact that it was bigger than the size 18s and 20s I had been buying, and I justified to myself, with a little help from the sales assistant, that it was a small make.

What was even more embarrassing was that I didn't realise what a difference the size of the person I was standing next to would make to how huge I looked. I learnt the hard way when I wore that outfit on the 1992 *Good Morning Australia* Christmas show. I'm a real glutton for punishment. It's not enough that I'm in a profession where you look bigger on camera (sadly television puts about 4 to 5 kilograms on you) but I made matters worse for myself on this particular occasion by standing next to the fabulously talented, but very tall and lean, Jeanne Little during the closing number of the show. You'll find two photos of the outfit in the picture gallery towards the middle of the book. One is with Jeanne and the *GMA* team and the other is with Bert and Matthew Newton.

Looking back at the photos taken when I was really big, they often show me partially hiding behind other people in an effort to conceal my body.

## So how do you get that shift in thinking?

Well if I knew what it took to permanently alter the chemicals in my brain so I always thought like a slim person instead of a fat person then I'd be a gazillionaire. Regrettably, I haven't figured that one out yet, and with such a lucrative fitness, health and weight-loss industry in Australia, estimated to turnover close to $7 billion annually, I'm not so sure greater minds than mine are actually working on a solution at this very minute. What I have learnt along the way is that I have to want to do it. I have to want to be thinner.

The old adage, 'You can lead a horse to water, but you can't make it drink', is very appropriate here. If I don't have the mind-set then there's no use anyone trying to help. And nagging only makes it worse, adding unnecessary pressure and angst. I knew that I had to start believing in myself and to keep telling myself that I could achieve it because if I didn't believe it, how could I expect anyone else to believe in me? There was no room for self-doubt.

## Leaving the past behind

As the years fly past and I physically age and look more mature on the exterior, I really don't feel that maturity on the interior. Mentally, I still feel like I'm in my thirties and I can quickly revert back much further to that scared fat little wog kid as my immediate emotional response when things frighten or confront me.

Making my inner child grow up and realising that I had to take an adult approach to handling the bad times was an important step, but it wasn't something that just came to me in my sleep. After much soul-searching, I realised that I couldn't change the past nor any of the traumatic things that had happened to me, especially in my childhood, so instead I made a deal with myself that I would change the way I reacted to them now that I was an adult.

For me this has been an extremely difficult but ultimately rewarding decision. While it's a decision I know I must continue to make on my own, I am certainly not alone and have sought lots and lots of guidance.

It hasn't been a smooth or even road to follow either and I've encountered lots of bumps, dead ends and sidetracks, with no shortage of tears and heartache. But I'm growing from these experiences and I think I've often learnt more from my failures.

'Even if you're on the right track, you'll get run over if you just sit there.'
- WILL ROGERS

It was time to finally confront my demons. In order to make my inner child grow up, I had to find out why I was reacting the way I did to certain stressful situations; and that meant I had to face my childhood traumas and come to terms with them.

This might be something that you feel you can't do on your own and if, like me, you feel you need to seek professional help then your GP is a great place to start.

I've made the same New Year's resolutions for a long as I can remember. They are: to work like I don't need the money, to love like I've never been hurt, to sing like no-one's listening, to dance like no-one's watching and there's another one that I'll have to leave to your imagination, but it relates to the 'unsealed' section of this book!

In the year 2000, leading up to the new millennium, I decided to add another resolution. I vowed that as I stepped into the twenty-first century, I was going to travel as light as possible mentally. To achieve this, I knew I couldn't take any excess emotional baggage with me. That meant anything traumatic that had happened to me in the previous century had to remain there. I gave myself permission to also leave behind the hurt, anxiety, blame, grief and all the other negative emotional feelings related to these traumas that would hinder my recovery in any way.

It wasn't easy to begin with, and it can still be extremely hard at times to stop myself from thinking about the sad, traumatic experiences, particularly when I'm alone and especially at night when I lay in bed trying to get to sleep and my mind starts to work overtime. It's a bit like when my tongue finds a rough spot on my tooth and despite my best intentions, I can't seem to keep myself from constantly coming back to it.

> 'We first make our habits and then our habits make us.'
> - JOHN DRYDEN

I had to learn to quickly recognise when the negative thoughts started creeping back into my mind and short-circuit them. I needed to train my brain to push them out of my head and into the past where they belonged and where I promised myself I would try and make them stay.

There are a few techniques I've picked up along the way to help me achieve this. I've learnt to put up a huge mental stop sign and use the four Rs that the fabulous Dr Jim suggested to me. Now when my mind drifts in a negative direction, I try not to allow it to impact on me nor to wallow in it for any length of time. You'll find out more about the four R's at the end of Chapter 5 'How do I say NO and mean it?'

My journey through the 'noughties' and onwards has been far more mentally enjoyable since I made that New Year's resolution to

STILL HALF MY SIZE

leave the past behind. While I draw on experiences from my past, I try to live very much in the present, and look positively into the future. To steal a line from a great Prince song, 'I now have to try and act my age and not my shoe size' when it comes to emotionally challenging situations.

## Baby steps

At my heaviest, the task of losing weight seemed like such an enormous one that I found it hard to see that there was even a light at the end of the tunnel. I was the size of two people but unfortunately I didn't get twice the brains to go with it, just twice the blubber. I couldn't remember ever being as big previously and the kilos were weighing heavily, not only on my bones but in my heart. It made me so depressed; I cried and cried until I didn't have any tears left.

They say that inside every fat person, there's a thin person trying to get out but in my case it seemed like there were two people cohabiting in there and I finally realised that there wasn't room for both of us. It was so daunting that it was very easy to convince myself that it was far too big a task, but I knew that was just another cop-out. Instead, I realised that by setting myself smaller, realistic goals, I was more likely to achieve them. I'd put the weight on one kilo at a time, therefore, the only way I could get it off was to do the same in reverse.

Making subtle changes to my life, especially my food fuel intake, meant that it didn't impact on me dramatically and it was easier to continue with these changes over a longer period of time. Yes, it did mean that the weight would come off more slowly, but for the first time I didn't feel like it was a race. One day at a time, one step at a time and one kilo at a time.

I was no longer obsessed with losing weight but instead with reducing my size, changing my shape and ultimately feeling good about myself. Basically I'm a pig, a glutton; I love food and plenty of it, so to starve myself on 'a diet' only made me miserable. It also made me feel hungry and think about food all the time so it was so easy to fall off the wagon.

Taking baby steps enabled me to not only set realistic, achievable goals but to still eat plenty of food and feel full. The food changes I have made are detailed in Chapter 3 'We are what we eat', which is also full of tips from my celebrity contributors.

I bumped into a male acquaintance of mine not so long ago who hadn't seen me for some time, and whose last visual image of me was when I was twice my size. He, like me, has been battling his weight forever, and his first response, after picking his jaw up from the ground in shock, was that I must have been starving myself. I assured him that it was quite the contrary; I now eat smaller portions and try and leave three hours between meals or two hours after a snack to eat again.

He went on to tell me how unhappy he was at still finding it impossible to lose weight. After a quick chat I discovered that he didn't have a sweet tooth, did a moderate amount of exercise and aside from a couple of beers each night and a few more on special occasions, he didn't think he was really doing the 'wrong thing'; but he couldn't seem to get any smaller. His job was physically taxing so any additional physical exercise wasn't an option for him.

We discussed what he was eating each day and he agreed to do a little baby steps experiment for me. He's a shiftworker and takes about a dozen bread rolls with him on every night shift and eats them at regular intervals while he's on duty. He said he couldn't cut down on the quantity as his work was quite strenuous and he needed that amount of food to give him the energy to complete his work tasks.

I discovered that he was filling each roll with lean meats and he was also spreading every roll with margarine. I asked him to do nothing else but eliminate all the unnecessary fat from his diet, and he said he didn't really eat fried foods.

When I suggested that he cut the margarine out altogether or substitute it, he said he'd tried before but found that the rolls were too dry. He didn't like mayonnaise, and as you'll see in Chapter 3 it is full of refined sugar, and he didn't like hummus or avocado either so instead I suggested adding tomato, which he said made the rolls too soggy. We compromised and he took the sliced tomato wrapped in cling wrap with him separately and added it to the rolls just before he ate them.

Without altering his exercise regime or reducing the quantity of food he was eating, he diligently eliminated all the unnecessary fat he'd been adding to his bread rolls and over the course of a few months he noticed for the first time that his waistline was decreasing. He was delighted that my baby steps approach had been successful for him as well. But as I've found out the hard way, it will only continue to work if he continues to do it. He needs to make it a lifestyle change. I've applied my baby steps approach to everything including my food intake, getting back into exercise and the goals I set for myself.

## Realistic goals

Being a size 22, I decided to set a realistic goal to get down to a size 14. Taking an overview of all my weight gains and losses over my lifetime I realised that the lowest I'd been able to get down to and maintain for any length of time was a size 14.

I'm sure one of the reasons why I hadn't been able to maintain my successful weight loss after the first time I went to Weight Watchers (WW) in the late 1970s, was because I didn't know when to stop shedding the weight.

I'd been so successful on the Weight Watchers program and steadily lost each week and reached my goal weight in record time, but I didn't stop there. Every Weight Watchers' leader who conducted their weekly meetings had to have had a weight problem and been trained through the WW program, so I should have listened to them.

Instead of taking their advice and implementing their maintenance program and being happy to control the size 12 that I had reached, I kept losing more weight and got down to a size 8–10. Everyone around me was telling me how fantastic I looked and I believed them. But that was all to be short-lived.

Well unfortunately not short enough to stop me from going out and buying heaps of tiny clothes and tight jeans. Ever noticed how many clothes you buy when you're that size and you hardly wear them because before you know it you can never get back into them? I'm really not meant to be that small, so it proved to be impossible to stay that way.

Before I knew it I had nibbled my way back to obesity and then continued to yoyo my way through life. Not only would I put back on all the weight I'd lost, but each time there'd be a few more kilos added.

The other reason I'd set a size 14 goal at the time was to help the hard-working team in Network Ten's wardrobe department. During the eight and a half years that I was on *Good Morning Australia* (1992–2000) with Bert Newton my dress size fluctuated from a size 16 when I started, all the way up to a size 20–22 and then back down to size 14.

Initially David Jones supplied my clothes and my lifesaver was Lissie Field, who's a brilliant freelance stylist now, but was then the head of wardrobe for Network Ten. Lissie would source clothes for me to wear on the show each week from the DJs racks and perform miracles to dress me, but it was getting more and more difficult the larger I became.

I'm such a hoarder and the majority of the smaller clothes that were in my wardrobe at home (which stretched between size 10 and size 20), were size 14 so I wanted to fit back into them and also to enable Lissie and I to go to just about any fashion label and have a good selection to choose from off the rack.

When I reached size 14 I was extremely happy and was feeling so much better about myself. Which then begs the age-old question: when you look good, do you feel good? Or the other way around: when you feel good, do you look good?

For the first time in more years than I could remember I was feeling both. I'd achieved my goal and I could now fit back into the majority of the clothes in my wardrobe. I became determined to maintain my new weight and never get any bigger so I continued with my lifestyle changes and they became a way of life.

It made me even prouder when I'd stayed a size 14 for over two years; never thinking that this long-term maintenance would result in me also going down another dress size. It was much to my surprise when I soon found I was down to a size 12 and not having any trouble maintaining that either.

By this stage I had cleared out all of the really big-size clothes in my wardrobe but I still couldn't part with many of the size 14 clothes that I really liked, just in case it really was the size I was meant to be. It wasn't until I had stayed a size 12 for about another two years that I took those favourite size 14 clothes and had them altered to fit me.

My dress size did fluctuate lower for a short time in 2001 when I went down to a size 8–10 after being heartbroken by a long-term relationship break-up, followed by bronchial pneumonia and then financial worries and all the stress that goes with these sorts of obstacles that we encounter along life's journey. But it didn't take me long to go back up to a more realistically sustainable dress size once I'd recovered.

## Compliments are great so long as you don't inhale them

I am not sure of the origin of the above saying, but it really caught my attention when I first heard someone in the television industry say it decades ago. I could relate to it well in relation to my work, having come across the odd person in the media who has an inflated ego juxtaposed to their talent. But it did take me a while to really understand and fully appreciate how much damage compliments could do to me in relation to my shape and size.

My interpretation of the saying is that when we inhale, the oxygen goes straight to our head and that's what compliments can do if we let them. Don't get me wrong, compliments are lovely to give and receive but I had to learn to put them in perspective. Everyone loves to tell you that you're looking slimmer, and we all love to hear it, but in the past it would sometimes trigger something in my brain that said, other people think I look good so I can relax and reward myself, stupidly with food. Unfortunately I wasn't in the right headspace to do that and simply just give myself a treat and then get back on the straight and narrow. Those treats would set off receptors in my brain that made them become too regular again and my old mind-set and eating habits would creep back, and of course so too would the weight.

While I can appreciate the heartfelt compliments that are often extended to me now, I am also still mindful of the horrible insults that were hurled at me by strangers when I was twice this size. I'm the only one who can ensure that I continue to get bouquets instead of brickbats. But as I am my greatest critic, being happy with myself is a much more important yardstick than any praise or criticism from others.

## Am I really hungry? The apple test

One of the lifestyle changes I realised that I had to make in order to shed weight and keep it off long-term was to stop using food for every reason other than if I was hungry.

It is always easy for me to find solace in food. And even easier to find an excuse to overeat: a social outing, a celebration or because I'm unhappy, bored, stressed, when I was premenstrual or simply out of habit. This time I had to break that cycle. I needed to work out how I could tell the difference between being physically hungry or just psychologically hungry.

That hasn't always been an easy thing to differentiate before so now I implement what I call the apple test. Whenever I crave food, I firstly check the clock to see if it's close to any meal times, in which case I could very well be physically hungry; if it hasn't been long enough since I last ate then I ask myself if I want an apple.

The reason I choose to do the apple test is because apples aren't my favourite food; I don't dislike them but they wouldn't be my first choice even when selecting between fruits. So if I'm looking for food to fill an emotional void, and I still do, then I generally find an apple won't achieve that for me. Therefore, I know that I'm not physically hungry and so instead of scouring the cupboards for something else to eat, as I've done too often in the past, I now distract myself mentally and go off and do things that are not related to food or have a big glass of water instead.

It's amazing how just taking your mind off food can make all the difference. Depending on the amount of time that I have to spare I either go for a walk, or give myself a facial, or ring a friend; anything that will distract my thoughts about food.

By the way, apples are one of the best fruits to eat because they have a low GI (glycaemic index), which in layman's terms is a measure of the effect a carbohydrate has on our blood glucose level.

## Keeping a diary

I've never been one to keep a journal or diary, even when I was young, and I have found it hard to maintain a travel log to record the wonderful memories and experiences I've enjoyed during overseas trips, so I wasn't impressed when I kept reading that I should keep a diary of what I'd eaten every day.

I'm not sure if you've ever kept a tally of everything that you've consumed in a day, but for a foodie like me it was an alarming exercise to say the least. The first time I did it I was too embarrassed to write down the 'bad' things that I had eaten and how much of them I'd consumed so I was very cryptic in my description just in case 'they' found it. And therefore 'those people' wouldn't be able to decipher what I'd eaten and discover my disgusting eating habits.

Deep down I knew that I could make sure that no-one around me was going to see my food logbook, but really I didn't want to admit to myself what I was consuming.

Of course, a blind man on a galloping horse could see the only person I was fooling was me. When I did finally wake up to myself, I wrote down everything that I ate and drank and in what quantities, as well as the exercise I did, and I even charted when my periods came and how long they lasted. I found the latter really important because as my hormones changed over the month, so too did my sweet cravings and binges. These hormonal changes became even more apparent when I went through menopause and you can read more in Chapter 7 'Managing the menopause madness'.

Keeping a food diary and a record of what exercise I did enabled me to have a blueprint from which to work. It gave me a much better overview of many aspects of my life and how they were affecting my weight. Armed with this knowledge I once again mentally took myself off to the moon to get a better handle on where I was going wrong and how I could improve.

## Read the label

I am now far more aware of everything that goes into my mouth and we are very lucky in Australia to have an industry-regulated code of practice in relation to the listing of all the contents of our food products. It has been mandatory since December 2002 for most packaged foods to include a nutrition panel that lists the energy level and the percentages of proteins, fats, sugars, carbohydrates, sodium (salt) etcetera inside. Other products simply list the ingredients in order of their quantity with the largest ingredient being listed first and then the other ingredients in order down to the smallest.

Some labelling can however be misleading especially when it comes to products that are 'low-fat' and I was keen to note the 'fat traps' that Danielle Teutsch pointed out in an article she wrote in the *Sun Herald* (2 February 2003). The biggest trap seems to be in savoury biscuits and crackers, which claim to be 90 per cent or 93 per cent fat-free. Food Standards Australia and New Zealand Managing Director Ian Lindenmayer was quoted as saying, 'The industry's code states that food less than 97 per cent fat-free should not be labelled fat-free.' He went on to say that a food actively promoted as being 90 per cent fat-free means it has 10 per cent fat, and that was not considered to be a low-fat product.

The article revealed that researchers at Deakin University found, after analysing foods and their low-fat equivalents, that in many cases the overall number of kilojoules was similar. The *Sun Herald* article cited an example of a brand of choc-chip cookies where there was 50 per cent less fat but only 6 per cent fewer kilojoules or calories. In some cases the fat-free products were no different from regular products. This study was led by Helen La Fontaine who points out that consumers believe these foods to be guilt-free and eat more, and it has been shown that people eat more after consuming a low-fat snack than a high-fat snack. When the fat is taken out, other ingredients that are as high or higher in energy usually replace it. Some low-fat item can be loaded up with very high amounts of sugars instead.

I've found it a good habit to read the nutrition panel on the side of the packaged foods that I buy and not just go by the fat-free label on the front. It alarmed me to learn that some brands of reduced-fat cow's milk and some soy milks have polyunsaturated oils added. Do you know what's in the food you're eating?

When you're reading the nutrition information panel, remember the packet size will vary so it's best to only use the 100 grams column when checking the contents and comparing products. For 'every day' foods it's recommended that the total fat is less than 10 grams. The saturated fat is less than 2 grams and sugar is less than 15 grams. Be sure to check which products also have less salt and more fibre.

Remember sugar has many different names including glucose, fructose, sucrose, dextrose, lactose, barley malt, corn syrup, fruit juice concentrate, maltodextrin, maltose, molasses, raw, crystal and brown sugar. On the food ingredient list, the closer sugar is to the beginning of the list, the more sugar the product contains.

In the nutritional panel, look for the 'carbohydrates (of which sugars)' figure to see how much sugar the product contains for every 100 grams.

In the United Kingdom, the National Health Service's guidelines have set more than 22.5 grams (5.4 teaspoons) of total sugars per 100 grams as high and 5 grams (1.2 teaspoons) of total sugars or less per 100 grams as low. An amount of sugars per 100 grams that is in between these figures is considered a medium level.

## No more diets!

There is a definite unhealthy mindset that I think we all get into if we talk about being 'on' or 'off' a diet and I'm not the only one who feels strongly about it. Scientists say women who diet to feel better about the way they look often feel depressed instead.

I remember reading an article in *The Sunday Telegraph* (29 December 2002) that said trying to lose weight could bring on a range of symptoms associated with clinical depression and anxiety. A study conducted by Aston University in England found that a preoccupation with food and the psychological stress of trying to lose weight led to impaired mental performance, as did changes to the diet itself.

Psychologists discovered that women on a diet showed poorer memory, slower reaction times, an inability to maintain attention and poorer planning ability than those not watching their weight. Dr Mike Green, a member of the study, explained that it was partly biological as dieters often cut out iron-rich foods, which reduces the flow of oxygen to the brain. However the major problem was that dieting is stressful and can lead to depression.

I recently learnt some more compelling facts about why diets don't work while reading 'The Genuine Article', a newsletter from the CEDRIC (Community Eating Disorder and Related Issues Counselling) Centre in Victoria, Canada.

CEDRIC defines disordered eating as a vicious circle of dieting followed by a binge and then incredible guilt and shame quickly followed by a new, improved diet. This becomes a way of life for many. The degree to which you feel guilt and shame around food, and how your body looks, is the degree to which you are a disordered eater. Michelle Morand from CEDRIC points out some scientific facts about what happens to your body when you diet.

Firstly your metabolism slows down. The problem with a low kilojoule diet is that it causes your body chemistry to undergo a fundamental change. Your body begins what's called a famine response. This is where your body believes that from now on, food could be very scarce. Instinctively your body changes to survive so it actively stores more of your consumed food as fat. As a result, even if you consume less food than you would normally, that food can be converted into body fat. It actually becomes decidedly harder to lose weight when your body's famine mechanism is in place.

This explains why in the past when I've starved myself I have either plateaued or barely made the needle move on those dreaded scales that I've now thrown away. My body was working against me.

There is good news: Michelle Morand points out that if you have messed up your metabolism to operate at the new, slower, fat-storing rate, it isn't permanent. While your metabolism is slow to change, you can get it back to its natural place just by not restricting your food fuel intake and by making sure you have a steady intake of food throughout the day so as not to trigger the famine response. And you can speed up your metabolism further by increasing your heart rate and I'll talk more about that in Chapter 4 'Get your motor running'.

I went on to read in 'The Genuine Article' that the average woman goes on over two diets a year and only one woman in 200 keeps any weight off for any reasonable length of time. That translates to 199 out of 200 women who are regularly engaging in a behaviour that decreases your self-esteem and body satisfaction, causes a negative change to your metabolism and possibly leads to eating disorders. All that torture and denial on a diet; without even getting any closer to the goal of physical acceptance!

Michelle Morand's article also highlighted another interesting statistic: a moderately active woman only needs approximately 250 fewer calories or 1045 kilojoules than a moderately active man.

How often have you watched your male friends with naturally healthy physiques eat whatever they like while you consume your celery and lettuce leaves? No prize for guessing whose 'diet' might be the problem.

At CEDRIC they advise if you are clinging to any of those dieting misconceptions to just stop and remind yourself that this is the diet mentality and that all it achieves is to keep you stuck in overeating. Let it go. Remember that compassion and self-trust are the keys. Trust that you are doing the best you can, and that that is enough.

## Don't let yourself get hungry

Being conscious that Mum had type 2 diabetes, as does my eldest brother Leon, instead of letting my blood sugar levels fluctuate too much by having big meals and then waiting too long between meals to feel hungry again, I now try to graze and eat smaller meals more regularly throughout the day.

Doing this also stops me from getting so hungry that despite all the arguments I have with myself, my 'balanced' diet ends up more like me eating food with both hands.

Arguing with myself always reminds me of a funny line I heard delivered by Kim Cattrall's character Samantha Jones in an episode of the television series *Sex and the City*, when she said, 'You'd go crazy if you tried to listen to all those little voices in your head.'

# Susie's ten steps to success

1. Don't weigh yourself

2. Let your clothes be the judge

3. Leave your past behind

4. Think positive

5. Take baby steps

6. Set realistic goals

7. Keep a food and beverage diary

8. Read the label

9. No more diets

10. Don't let yourself get hungry

# CHAPTER 3

# WE ARE WHAT WE EAT

n order to finally look at my body objectively I had to disassociate it from my heart. I decided I had to make my body a separate entity or object that I could focus on and look after like a treasured possession that I valued rather than just taking it for granted. One of my closest friends refers to her body as a temple but every time I think of temples my first thought is always of the movie *Indiana Jones and the Temple of Doom*! Fantastic movie as it was, it's not a good image to immediately associate with your body, so I looked farther afield.

An analogy that I could relate to better was a motor vehicle. My dad had two service stations and I know a little bit about cars so I found it easy to make the comparisons between a car and my body.

## Become your dream car

Ever since I was knee-high to a grasshopper, my dream car has always been a sleek and sexy red Mercedes convertible. So far I've only been able to afford the red convertible part, when I owned a fabulous little Ford Capri.

Our dream car can be just that – whatever we dream of – and I'd love you to do this little exercise with me.

Start by choosing any make of car you think best resembles the dream car you'd be proud to drive your mind around in through the rest of your life's journey. In this case, as it's all imaginary, money is no object. The model of your dream car is already determined by the year you were born.

Now I want you to imagine what sort of vehicle would best describe your current size and shape.

How far is it from looking like your dream car?

What changes in your shape will get your current chassis to start resembling your dream car?

Is there too much 'junk in the trunk'?

Is your upholstery bulging out from around middle of your seats?

Or is your engine the part that's giving you trouble; maybe it's just not humming along smoothly under your bonnet?

I went through a lot of vehicle changes before I could finally reached by dream car size and shape.

When I was carrying 50 plus kilos more than I am now I felt like an eighteen-wheel semitrailer that needed a six-lane highway to get around on, but as soon as I dropped a couple of dress sizes I felt much more compact and thought I looked more like a five-door people mover.

When I reached size 14 I was delighted that my body had now turned into a sedan but I still felt a bit chunky, like my old Datsun 180B. I turned into a variety of sedans over quite a few years as I toned up my size 14 frame before finally getting down to a size 12 and reaching my dream car size and shape.

Since 2005 I haven't always managed to drive my dream car around and have found myself back in a sedan, especially in the cooler months, and turning into that people mover a couple of times since.

More tweaking was needed and the most recent changes to my food fuel mix have enabled me to get back down to a size 12 again, and even take the top down in my red Mercedes sports car. You might go through a variety of vehicles too before you reach your dream car size and shape.

Carrying extra kilos can be ageing and if you want to look like you've wound back the odometer then start setting your sights on becoming your dream car.

While it's always tempting to go for the most expensive car, like a Lotus or a flashy Ferrari or Lamborghini, be more realistic when selecting your vehicle because like your body, you want one that you can handle comfortably, you'd be proud to be seen around in and one that can go the distance without requiring an unrealistic amount of time-consuming upkeep, or any trips to the panel beaters in order to maintain it to assembly line specs.

Once you've pragmatically chosen your dream car and you know what vehicle you currently most resemble, you can formulate very visual goals that need to be achieved to succeed.

## Food fuel

Regardless of how well you service your car or take care of it, one thing's for sure, no vehicle can run without fuel and neither can our bodies. Years ago when we had super and standard petrol, if you put the wrong one in your car it would 'ping' and backfire. While your car would still run on it, it wouldn't be performing at its best and consistently filling it with incorrect or inferior gas would certainly damage the engine in the long term.

I would never deliberately put the wrong fuel into my car yet for most of my life I've constantly been putting the wrong fuel into my body and overfilling it as well, but I'll address the overeating part of my problem a little later.

My analogy doesn't always have identical parallels. It's much easier not to overfill a car with petrol. These days the fuel tanks in cars and nozzles on bowsers vary in size, depending if it's petrol or diesel or E10, to hopefully eliminate the chance of putting the wrong fuel into it. Unfortunately, it isn't nearly as easy to avoid these mistakes when fuelling our body. There are so many variables that can come into play when I'm in total control of what ingredients I put into the cocktail of fuel for my body.

# Choose the best mix of fuel for your body

The quantity and the quality of your fuel intake can vary enormously from day to day and ultimately the choice of what goes into your mouth is yours.

The fuel for your dream car is provided by food and the energy is measured in calories or kilojoules (1 calorie = 4.2 kilojoules). The amount of energy you're planning to expend while driving your body around throughout the day will then determine how much you'll need to adjust your fuel intake accordingly.

If you are constantly overfilling your body or loading it up with high-energy fuel and not burning a bit of rubber in return then you can probably expect to develop a spare tyre, generally around your waist, in addition to the one that's probably already over-inflating in your boot.

And while you'll be able to notice the shape of your chassis changing, there's also the extra wear and tear that's constantly being placed on all the components of your body by carrying the extra load, like the discs in your spine and your knees, which would equate to the shock absorbers or struts in your car.

Likewise, if you underfill your body then you'll trigger the famine response, which is described in detail in the previous chapter, and if the fuel is inferior then you're depriving your body of the important nutrients it needs to run at peak performance. You'll notice that you start to feel sluggish and run out of energy quicker, and if you're constantly running your body tank near empty, then this can also lead to long-term internal damage and reduce the number of kilometres you're going get on your body clock.

There are guidelines issued by governments the world over as to what constitutes a healthy intake of fuel, but remember that you're unique and your dream car has been custom-made, which means there is no other vehicle the same anywhere in the world. Therefore, you'll need to customise your fuel to suit your make and model as well as your individual lifestyle.

Nutritionists advise women who are overweight to adjust the total energy value of foods that are fuelling their bodies to no less than 1500 calories (6300 kilojoules) daily if you wish to release your excess fat stores. Men can have a slightly higher energy intake of 1800 calories (7560 kilojoules) per day. Energy comes from these sources:

**Carbohydrates:** complex or simple (low and high octane) 4 calories (almost 17 kilojoules) per gram.

**Protein:** animals or vegetable based 4 calories (almost 17 kilojoules) per gram.

**Fats:** monounsaturated, saturated, polyunsaturated, hydrogenated trans fats (leaded and unleaded fuel) 9 calories (almost 38 kilojoules) per gram.

**Alcohol:** 7 calories (29 kilojoules) per gram.

Each of these foods is converted into glucose at varying rates to fuel the body. If you grew up, like me, being taught all about the food pyramid, which recommends that cereals and grains be the biggest amount of your fuel intake and then fruit and vegetables and that fats be the least, then your energy source would most likely be around 70 per cent carbohydrates, 15 per cent protein and 15 per cent fat.

The American Diabetes Association recommends 60 per cent carbohydrates, 20 per cent protein and 20 per cent fat.

Barry Sears PhD, who co-wrote *The Zone – A Dietary Road Map* with Bill Lawren, believes 40 per cent carbohydrates, 30 per cent protein and 30 per cent fat is the favourable mix.

Sitting in the driver's seat, you are in complete control and it's often a matter of trial and error until you find the food fuel mix that gives you your best performance and it is important to constantly monitor and adjust the mix and your intake.

## Carbohydrates – high- and low-octane fuel

Let's start with carbohydrates (commonly abbreviated to carbs), which include fruits, vegetables, cereals, bread, pasta, rice, dairy products and sugar.

In Dr Sears's *The Zone*, he explains that we need a continual intake of carbs; however any carbs not immediately used by the body will be stored in the form of glycogen in the liver and the muscles. The bad news is they don't have much storage space so any excess carbohydrates are then converted into fat and stored in the fatty tissue. *The Zone* also points out that your brain devours around two-thirds of the carbohydrates circulating in the bloodstream but the brain can't access the carbs stored in your muscles, only in your liver.

Carbohydrates come in two forms: simple and complex, or as I call them, the high- or low-octane components of our food fuel. Aside from its energy measurement, each carbohydrate also has a glycaemic index rating or GI. This is a measure of carbohydrates based on their immediate effect on blood glucose levels. Some carbohydrates break down easily during digestion such as sugar, glucose, sweets, as well as highly processed foods such as white bread and biscuits. They have a high GI-rating, which can give you a rapid energy boost but can also make your energy levels plummet just as quickly when this energy is spent.

Other carbohydrates break down slower and are released into the bloodstream gradually and therefore have a low GI-rating such as apples, stone fruits, grapes, oranges, sweet potato, pasta, corn, and sourdough, rye and wholemeal breads. Legumes or pulses such as lentils, chickpeas and beans (including baked, mung, kidney, haricot and butter) are also all low GI.

It's good to monitor your activity levels and balance your low and high-GI carbs accordingly. If you know you are going to be revving your engine and going around the block a few times today then you can indulge in a mixture of high and low-GI carbs, because you know you're going to be burning them off.

Alternatively, if you know that you are not going to get your motor much past idling then favouring low-GI carbs will help maintain a steady blood-sugar level and control the amount of the hormone insulin that the pancreas secretes into the bloodstream. Dr Barry Sears goes onto explain in *The Zone* that essentially insulin is a storage hormone, evolved to put aside excess carbohydrate calories in the form of fat in case of future famine. So eating too many carbs is sending a message to the body's fatty tissue, via the insulin, to store fat and not to release any stored fat either. This makes it virtually impossible for you to use your own stored body fat for energy, so these excess fat-free carbs in your food can not only make you gain unwanted fat, they also make sure you retain that fat.

I've sourced all the GI-ratings I mention in this book from *The New Glucose Revolution* by Professor Jennie Brand-Miller, Kaye Foster-Powell and Associate Professor Stephen Colaguiri (Hodder). My knowledge expanded a great deal more during a TV interview I did with Professor Brand-Miller, who has a great way of explaining complex things simply that we can all understand.

The glycaemic index was first developed in 1981 by Dr David Jenkins, a professor of nutrition at the University of Toronto, Canada primarily to determine which foods were best for people with diabetes.

Mum was a member of Diabetes Australia and was very impressed with all the information she was sent regularly on the latest research on diabetes. Mum's insulin dependence was the catalyst for her to live low GI, in order to control her sugar levels and not gain excess weight. There's no doubt when I consciously eat fewer high-octane carbs I am not hungry between meals.

The good news is that not all your carbs need to be low GI. If you add some low-octane fuel to each meal that will help moderate the high-GI foods to a medium-GI level.

Even though most fruits are low-octane, they accelerate to high-octane quickly when juiced. The reason is that you're removing the fibre, which is the non-digestible part of the carbohydrate. More fibre means it will take longer for your blood-sugar level to rise and in turn your pancreas will need to release less insulin into your bloodstream.

Also, the more fibre you add to your fuel mix, the better your muffler will run. Fibre also clears out your exhaust pipes giving you a much more comfortable ride, and at the same time helps you to obtain or retain your dream-car shape.

The latest medical research reveals that fibre is the hero to having good gut health and Dr Maxwell Strong explains why in Chapter 8 'Twenty-first century discoveries'.

# Sugar addiction

The most damaging component of our food fuel is the excessive amount of glucose we consume.

The best car analogy I can make is when we ingest too much sugar in our food fuel and it goes through our blood stream, it's like putting a corrosive in our gas tank that will start rusting the fuel line and damage all the parts as it flow through the engine and the rest of the car's mechanics.

There is plenty of medical evidence around now that clearly shows how addictive sugar is, in fact, QUT and the University of Queensland led a world-first study in 2016 that shows Food & Drug Administration (FDA) approved prescription drugs currently used to successfully treat nicotine addiction, can work the same way when it comes to sugar cravings. (www.qut.edu.au/health/about/news/news?news-id=103304)

*The American Journal of Clinical Nutrition* released the findings of a study back in 1995 that showed the use of an opiate blocker, successful in treating heroin addicts, reduced the consumption of sweet, high-fat foods in obese and lean female binge eaters. (ajcn.nutrition.org/content/61/6/1206.abstract)

Instead of us taking these sorts of drugs to control our sugar cravings wouldn't it be easier and better for our health if we just cut out the hidden sugars in our foods? Or at least reduced them substantially?

This was the first of many questions I put to Dr Gary Fettke and Pete Evans in order to learn more about the best food fuel we should adopt.

**Dr Gary Fettke:** The important issue is educating the individual on the effects of added sugars and how they affect behaviour and health. I see the community awareness has improved dramatically over the last few years. Once informed, you can make choices. Many still will not but then we still have people smoking despite the warnings.

**Pete Evans:** I always recommend working with your healthy health professional (if you can find one these days) when changing your diet, and when considering sugar we need to realise that a low-carbohydrate diet coupled with a cyclical ketogenic approach is what the researchers are now advising as the optimal way to be fuelling our bodies for health and longevity.

You may wish to ask your readers to read Dr Joseph Mercola's book titled *Fat for Fuel* for further reading. When people think about sugar they think about the white stuff whereas we need to be thinking from a blood sugar point of view in the body, so cutting our high-carb foods like potatoes, rice, bread (even if it is wholegrain, it makes no difference) as all of these foods raise the blood sugars in people so we need to minimise that, which is why a low-carb paleo approach is the key. Low carb in itself doesn't work for the majority because they are still including dairy, which is inflammatory to our bodies, so go the next step and go low-carb paleo!

**Susie:** Staggeringly, an Australian gets diagnosed with type 2 diabetes every five minutes. Almost two million Australians have already been identified, with around another million estimated to be living with it undiagnosed. Medical experts have dubbed type 2 diabetes as the silent pandemic of the twenty-first century.

Dr Gary, what is fructose? And why can it be so harmful?

**Dr Gary Fettke:** Fructose is half of sugar. Combined with glucose it makes sucrose which we know commonly as sugar. Glucose and fructose are the basic forms of carbohydrate but are metabolised very differently. Fructose is also found in similar percentages in honey and high fructose corn syrup.

Fructose tends to be naturally available in seasonal fruit and in nature is consumed in quantities that can be stored by animals as fat for winter hibernation.

The problem in society is that 'we' are eating it to excess every day. That unnatural excess tends to be involved in driving behaviour as well as being deposited as fat in our livers and then around the body.

Fructose is involved in other metabolic pathways involving raising blood pressure, obesity, type 2 diabetes, and hunger and lipoprotein storage ('bad' cholesterol-sized particles).

Small amounts are naturally occurring. But if taken to excess over a long time the effects accumulate.

**Susie:** Can we reverse this diabetes tsunami by just eating the right food, and of course education?

**Dr Gary Fettke:** Yes. The complications of type 1 and type 2 diabetes are completely avoidable with a low-carbohydrate lifestyle.

**Pete Evans:** When it comes to type 2 diabetes, yes we can not only prevent type 2 diabetes from happening but we can reverse it in the majority of cases through correct nutrition as well as factoring in the other pillars of wellness such as sleep, emotional wellbeing, adequate sunlight exposure, the cleanest water as well as the simple act of moving our bodies in a nourishing way.

**Susie:** The World Health Organization (WHO) has dropped its sugar intake recommendations from 10 per cent of our daily calorie intake to 5 per cent after releasing draft guidelines and encouraging public comment in 2014.

For an average adult that equates to about six teaspoons or 25.2 grams of sugar per day, which is easy to measure if you're spooning sugar into a cup of tea or coffee but there is an unhealthy amount of 'hidden' sugar in processed foods, according to the WHO.

To put it in perspective, a single can of soft drink may contain up to sixteen teaspoons or 67.2 grams of sugar, which is close to three times the recommended daily sugar allowance. There is one teaspoon (4.2 grams) of sugar in every tablespoon of most tomato and barbecue sauces and that can more than double in sweet chilli sauce. There can be up to a whopping ten teaspoons of sugar (42 grams) in two thin slices of some supposedly healthy wholegrain bread, which is horrifying in itself and even worse when compared to a chocolate bar with 8.5 grams (just over two teaspoons) of sugar.

If you want to check other foods, David Gillespie, author of *Sweet Poison – Why Sugar Makes Us Fat* has a free food ready-reckoner on his website www.howmuchsugar.com. His database has over 2000 foods (not brand specific) showing the amount of fructose and omega-6 fat in those foods.

**Susie:** Is it time for us to put warning labels on these pre-packaged foods like we do on cigarettes?

**Dr Gary Fettke:** I would like to see us improve our labels but acknowledge that they are a lot better than many other places around the world. Imagery will have an effect for many.

I think a sugar tax, even a small one raises awareness and acknowledges that governments see our sugar and processed-food consumption as a health issue.

**Pete Evans:** I think people just need to be aware of what real food is, and people will still eat junk food regardless of if there is a label on it, just like people still smoke even though there are labels on the cigarettes now. It comes down to education but the right type of education, as the one we have now that all schools, hospitals and aged care centres use is completely wrong and is damaging the health of the population.

**Susie:** Could we find a simple, visual way of showing how much sugar (carbohydrates), salt and fat is in each product and use the red, amber, green background to indicate at a glance how many times they are over the recommended daily intake and at least let the buyer be aware?

**Dr Gary Fettke:** An image-based sugar symbol would be beneficial. However, we have the health star rating system in now that was endorsed by the food industry. It is being manipulated and creating, more, rather than less confusion in the community.

**Pete Evans:** Again it would depend on what the person has eaten in their whole day, and I will go back to basics again and focus on eating an abundance of lower carb veggies with some higher ones on the plate in small amounts, then add some well sourced animal protein and fat from land or sea animals and cook it or drizzle it in good fats.

**Susie:** Surely the Big Food industry as a whole should be held accountable for manufacturing these extremely unhealthy products. It's a multi-billion dollar industry so these companies won't be in a hurry to change their contents, especially if their customers no longer enjoy the taste. Is there anything we as consumers can do to make them start to change and improve the contents inside? Or is not buying these pre-packaged foods simply the only way to go?

**Dr Gary Fettke:** I firmly believe in a revolution led by the people, the consumers with buying power. The people see the benefit of reducing sugar and processed food straight away. That is working now. Waiting on a top-down approach from government when they are influenced by lobbyists is a long way off. We cannot wait.

**Pete Evans:** Sorry to sound like a broken record but it is not the food manufacturers' fault. You can't blame an alcohol maker who makes vodka for someone's demise through drinking, a known poison, the same can be said for cigarettes, as no-one is forcing people to drink alcohol or smoke, so the same can be said for food manufacturers, they are just responding to consumer demand. I for one do not give them any of my hard earned dollars, which is why paleo is not the favoured approach for many industries as we basically make them redundant when people choose to love themselves through the food or beverages they consume. We need to stop blaming and instead we need to take responsibility for our own actions and thrive.

**Susie:** When I stopped eating refined sugars, bad fats and refined carbohydrates like pasta and bread, my sugar cravings disappeared.

It also created a positive domino effect for me; including calibrating my tastebuds to once again appreciate just how sweet whole fruit and vegetables do taste, finding I'm not as hungry so I'm not eating as much, I'm feeling and being more energetic and as a visual reward: a reduction in my size and shape.

**Susie:** How can we expect our willpower to hold, when food manufacturers spend a fortune employing scientists and chemists, whose sole purpose is to find the bliss point (the perfect combination of sugar, salt and fat) that makes us crave the food more, instead of it satisfying us?

**Dr Gary Fettke:** It keeps coming back to understanding how processed food affects you as well as how the marketing of 'junk' is there to distract you. We also have a culture of eating for pleasure rather than survival. To make changes for your health many need SAM in their life: support, accountability and motivation. Finding someone to go that journey with you makes the difference.

**Pete Evans:** It is simple – don't fucken buy that crap. End of story…they are not forcing you to eat it!!!

You can read the rest of Pete Evans and Dr Gary Fettke's interviews at the end of this chapter.

## Why do I crave fat?

The foods that have a high percentage of fat in them are also deadly for me when it comes to turning my sleek and sexy convertible back into a one-tonne truck with extra boot space.

While I know the psychologists' eternal debate of nature versus nurture will continue indefinitely, in the case of craving fat, it can now be directly attributed to nature.

I watched a brilliant program on TV called *Human Nature,* which explained that our craving for fat can be traced back to caveman days. Being a primate who didn't swing through the trees, when food was scarce humans survived longer if they had fat stored and that's why we have much larger buttocks than apes.

That would explain, according to research conducted in 2005 by scientists at the University of Burgundy in France, why there is a protein on the tip of our tongue that craves fat.

I'm grateful that I don't live in an era where I have to hunt for my food and there's no doubt, compared to cavemen we're all living a much more sedentary lifestyle with a lot more fat-enriched foods from which to choose.

I've often wonder what evolution will need to take place to compensate for the dramatic unhealthy changes the majority of the Western world has made to our diet and lifestyle, for us to survive long term as a species on this planet.

## Crave Man article

There's a fabulous article written by a *Washington Post* staff writer on 27 April 2009 entitled 'Crave Man' that you can easily access online. It details the lengths that Harvard-trained doctor David A Kessler went to in order to understand a problem that has plagued him since his childhood of obesity: why certain foods are impossible to resist.

He even climbed into huge dumpsters and dug through the garbage in order to retrieve the ingredients label on the empty packets from his favourite restaurant chain, information they'd declined to provide when requested. He details his findings, which are starling, in his book, *The End of Overeating*. Instead of satisfying our hunger, the sugar-fat-salt combo stimulates the brain to crave more.

Dr Kessler was appointed by President George W Bush to investigate the tobacco industry and he sees parallels between the tobacco and food industries. He says, 'Both are manipulating consumer behaviour to sell products that can harm health.'

## You never see a fat sheep in a drought

When I thought about it in the context of sheep and drought, it wasn't hard to realise that where food is generally very plentiful in countries like Australia, New Zealand and America, that's also where a large percentage of the population has a weight problem. And I am one of those people.

As an omnivore there were too many food choices and when push came to shove I'd more often than not opt for the fattening alternative. It's clear to me now that my body runs at its optimum on Dr Gary Fettke's LCHF Low Carbohydrate Healthy Fats food fuel (full details at the end of this chapter) but back then I had to find a way to permanently reduce the amount of unhealthy fats in my diet to begin with; it was like lead and weighing me down.

# Fats – leaded and unleaded fuel

For years I'd fallen prey to the popular notion that low-fat alternatives were always better for you to eat than the full-fat version and I'm the first to say how misled I was. I've highlighted earlier what happens when the fat is taken out to make a fat-free or reduced-fat version and it's generally filled up with harmful levels of sugar instead.

I've categorised the fats in our food fuel as either leaded or unleaded. Dietary fat contains more than double the amount of kilojoules (energy) per gram than carbohydrate so it needs to be consumed in moderation (there's the M word again).

Leaded fats should be limited and in some cases avoided; including some saturated fats like the skin of a chicken, margarines and vegetable shortening. Artificial trans fats or hydrogenated fats are fats that have been saturated with hydrogen to turn them from a liquid into a solid and may be hidden in baked goods as well as processed foods, snack foods, fried foods, fast foods, chocolate, pizza dough and tubs of ice cream. Be sure to read labels when you shop.

The 2015 Guidelines for Americans recommend keeping trans and saturated fats to less than 10 per cent of your daily calories, or no more than roughly one-third to one-half of your total fat consumption, with your goal to consume as close to zero grams of trans fat as possible.

I'm not talking about the low-fat or reduced-fat varieties of the full-fat equivalent when I describe unleaded fats or healthy fats. Healthy unleaded fats include monounsaturated vegetable oils, such as canola, peanut or olive oil. Nuts and seeds are rich in healthy fats, and make a better alternative in your salad than cheese. Avocados and fish such as salmon, herring and mackerel, provide plenty of healthy fats to help leave you feeling sated after a meal.

Dr Gabe Mirkin, who has authored and co-authored over a dozen books on health, fitness and sports medicine including *The Healthy Heart Miracle* approaches eating and fitness in terms of a healthy heart rather than a smaller jean size and points out that no matter what size or shape you are, these 'leaded' fats can tend to raise blood cholesterol and increase your risk of heart disease. The only way to cut back or eliminate partially hydrogenated fats (the source of trans fats) from your diet is to read the label of every processed food you buy. Scan through the list of ingredients and if it contains the words 'partially hydrogenated', Dr Mirkin advises to put it back on the shelf.

Most of us find that almost impossible to do, as these unhealthy fats can be found in most pre-packaged foods. When you can't avoid these foods altogether choose the ones with the least amount of saturated or trans fats in them.

Dr Mirkin also points out that it's much harder when you eat out, because you have no way to tell what's going on in the kitchen. Fast-food restaurants and chains use a lot of pre-prepared frozen foods that they reheat for you. These are usually loaded with partially hydrogenated fats. Dr Mirkin says you're safer at restaurants that prepare your food from scratch.

Asian restaurants use oils, not margarine or shortening. Most French restaurants use huge amounts of butter, which Dr Mirkin agrees is better than trans fats but not great if you're trying to lose weight or control cholesterol. Italian, Greek, Spanish and other Mediterranean restaurants tend to use the much healthier option of olive oil.

## Why I became a vegetarian

I often get asked why I became a vegetarian and if it was for any ethical or moral reasons. The short answer is no. While I vehemently oppose the illegal poaching of wild animals, and the clubbing of baby seals horrifies me beyond belief, I have no issue if an animal is bred in captivity for its food or its coat so long as it's raised in a clean and healthy environment and then slaughtered as quickly and humanely as possible.

In the mid-1980s my weight was out of control again and I realised that I needed to seriously look at the fuel I was putting into my body. I'd repeatedly put myself through the misery of eating skinless chicken breasts when all I really wanted was the skin, the bum (parson's nose) and the wings, which as we know are all the really bad fatty bits.

The best tasting part of a T-bone steak or chop for me is the cooked fat that runs down one side and it was always torture cutting it off and throwing it away and only eating the meat. My preference was always for fatty juicy pork or beef spare ribs or only eating the crackling and none of the roast pork. No matter how much apple sauce you smothered over grilled pieces of new-fashioned lean pork it didn't seem to improve in flavour.

This led me to decide, some might say with pretzel logic, that if I couldn't continue to eat all these bad but yummy fatty bits that I loved and if my willpower was always being challenged and I would feel miserable every time I had to throw these bits away in the bin, just to eat the rest of the meat that I didn't enjoy as much, then I'd be better off abstaining from eating it altogether.

It was a big decision to make a total lifestyle change and become a vegetarian. That meant no more meat, no more chicken, no more fish or seafood. When I'd made the mental commitment to abstain from eating these altogether, it was actually easier to say 'No' upfront rather than to put myself through the torment finding the inner strength each time I had to discard the yummy tasting high-fat parts. For me the pressure was off because I had eliminated the temptation altogether.

Luckily, my GP Dr Jim had been a vegetarian for more decades than he'd probably care to admit and he gave me lots of guidance.

He explained to me that one of the big mistakes so many people, especially teenage girls, make when they decide to become a vegetarian is they simply eliminate the proteins such as meat, fish, eggs, and cheese from their food fuel mix. And if you don't replace the foods that are high in iron, like red meat, with alternative vegetarian proteins such as pulses, beans or nuts then you can develop all sorts of health issues, especially with women who are menstruating.

Women need the iron to replace what we lose in our blood during every monthly period. When we remove these iron-rich foods and don't replace it with any other iron-rich foods then it's easy to become anaemic and lethargic, which can then develop into more serious health problems. It also means that you'll tend to eat far too many carbs instead. It's the fat in the protein that makes us feel full.

By the way, iron is extremely hard to absorb into our body so I learnt that if you are eating iron-rich foods, have something high in vitamin C like orange juice or chew vitamin C tablets with it and it will help your body absorb more of the iron into your system.

A lot of people take iron tablets; I find them to be very constipating, so if I'm feeling that my body engine is sluggish and hard to start first thing in the morning, or I'm feeling weary, then I'll take a course of liquid iron, which is available at most health-food stores. I store it in the fridge.

I decided not to be too radical in my approach to becoming a vegetarian and remove too much calcium-enriched foods from my food fuel to begin with and run the risk of long-term problems such as osteoporosis.

Instead of becoming totally vegan – that's where you eat no animal products or bi-products whatsoever – I opted for the softer alternative of being a lacto-ovo vegetarian, which still left milk, yoghurt, eggs and cheese (more on cheese later) for my protein and calcium.

It now became easier to control my food fuel intake and especially the high-fat component and as a result I began to shed the weight again.

## The other luxuries I couldn't afford to eat

While being a vegetarian was helping me reach my dream-car goal at meal times, I was still falling back into old bad behaviours, especially comfort eating, and as a result I went back to filling myself with unhealthy snacks. Before I knew it my weight started to yo-yo again.

I was feeling unhappy navigating around in a body shape resembling a Toyota HiAce people mover rather than the sports car I'd longed to be.

It was back to the drawing board; I kept an honest logbook of my fuel intake and if my speedo was clocking up any exercise.

Clearly I had to implement a few more lifestyle changes and get my food fuel correct if I were to succeed long term.

It became very apparent that I enjoyed putting things starting with the letter 'C' into my mouth most of all and they seem to be the things that always got me into the most trouble, like chocolate, cheese and chips.

I'd been to see a naturopath and she suggested that I give up anything with yeast in it for a while to help another problem I was experiencing, so I figured if I had to give up bread and cheese then I'd bite the bullet and give up chocolate at the same time.

I think I lasted a couple of years not eating any grains but I haven't eaten hard cheese since 1995 and I lasted around fifteen years not eating any chocolate whatsoever.

The cornerstone of my ongoing success today is to keep a watchful eye on the amount of refined sugar and grains that I'm consuming in my food fuel mix and to make sure I'm eating enough protein.

I found out firsthand that it's not easy to be a 'healthy vegetarian' and keep the weight off, especially when you want to eat out. In my experience, most vegetarian options are generally overflowing with complex carbohydrates like pasta or rice and most often, the only protein on offer is high-fat cheese and the dish is habitually smothered in it.

## How much lead should I have in my fuel?

The hardest word in the English language for me to actually master in life is 'moderation'. I'm an 'all or nothing' girl and my closest friend, also Susie, sums me up best as having a 'flair for excess'. This becomes immediately apparent whenever I get the taste of cheese or chocolate.

I love cheese and never found it difficult to devour large slabs of it, no matter what sort: blocks of tasty cheese, blue vein, camembert, you name it! And I couldn't just stop at one wafer-thin slice either.

I'm sure I'm not the only one guilty of demolishing an entire cheese and fruit platter after dinner in a restaurant or making inroads into the cheese and biscuits at a party. There's one thing that makes cheese taste even yummier to me, and that's when the cheese is melted. Pizzas were high on my fast foods list and if I had friends pop by I'd be a big hit when I'd serve up taco dip with lots and lots of melted cheese on top and corn chips.

Eating all of that again would guarantee my sports car would start turning into a chock-a-block full station wagon.

Until I gave up cheese, I hadn't noticed how prominent cheese is on restaurant menus, often being the only vegetarian alternative, and just how much cheese is added to takeaway foods.

Recently I was excited to see a new salad bar open up close to me but was soon disappointed to discover that out of about a dozen spectacular looking salads, there were only a couple that didn't have either grated cheese or meat all through them or they were smothered in dressing. I tried eating low-fat cheese but it didn't really have much of an impact because even these cheeses were still far too high in fat to be consumed in such high quantities.

For instance, in a 30-gram serve of cheddar cheese there is a whopping ten grams of saturated fat and 120 calories (500 kilojoules). If you're like me and not a 'metric baby' then 30 grams equates to one ounce or two tablespoons

According to the Institute of Medicine, the percentage of calories in our food fuel that should be from fat is 20 to 35 per cent. For example, if you eat 2000 calories (8200 kilojoules) a day, 400 calories (1640 kilojoules) to 2850 kilojoules (700 calories) should be from fat, which equals 44 to 78 grams of fat daily.

The 2010 Dietary Guidelines for Americans suggest obtaining less than 10 per cent of our daily calories from saturated and trans fat.

Whatever way you want to calculate, it's just a couple of bite-size morsels to me. I'd use at least 120 grams of cheese when making an open grilled sandwich to ensure I'd get a thick, even layer that came to the edges of my bread and melted over the sides so the crusts wouldn't burn. That snack alone had 40 grams of fat, which is close to my maximum daily fat allowance and more than twice the recommended intake of saturated fats.

Just half-filling my sandwich maker with one of my favourite combos, it was easy to use half a camembert and a small avocado. The cheese has around 25 grams of fat, the avocado 15 grams, not to mention the two or three tablespoons of margarine (12 grams of fat per tablespoon) that I'd use to on the outside of the bread to make the jaffles well toasted and crisp. So let's conservatively say its 76 grams of fat, despite the fact that I know how heavy-handed I can be. That little snack totals more than the recommended fat intake for two days.

It soon became apparent that cheese was a part of my food fuel that wasn't compatible with the smooth running of my Mercedes sports car and being able to take the top down in summer. As I wasn't prepared to size up to a sedan or get larger upholstery, I chose instead not to fill my dream car with cheese.

It doesn't mean that you can't still enjoy your sandwich maker but now try some unleaded fillings, like creamed corn, baked beans, tomato and avocado instead of the cheese. Try leaving off the margarine or butter altogether and spray the bread with a thin film of olive-oil spray and your jaffles sandwich will still toast and brown up without all the fat.

## Chocolate

My worst food addiction is, without a doubt, chocolate. I've already fessed up to eating three entire packets of eleven Tim Tams (5 grams of fat per biscuit) in one go, and more than once. But that's just the tip of the iceberg.

My love of chocolate wasn't just limited to Tim Tams. I've been asked by a few magazines over the years what job I'd love to do if I wasn't in media and my immediate reply has always been a chocolate taster for my favourite Swiss chocolate company Lindt; and everyone thinks I'm kidding!

It's scary when you know every Cadbury's Roses chocolate by their wrapper. And Easter was like a bushman's picnic for me. If I had to choose a 'last meal' it would definitely include a jumbo block of Cadbury's milk chocolate.

While I don't think I could give Lard-Ass, the pie-eating champion in the movie *Stand by Me* a run for his money, I did win an eating competition of sorts. It was around 1992 when I was working for Capital Television and their office in Wollongong was opposite the most delicious gourmet food store. On occasions a couple of us would walk across for a mid-morning treat. This particular day as we looked into the glass cabinet, we saw the chef placing the yummiest looking freshly made mud cake on the top shelf so we decided on a piece each. When he cut the slices I noticed how thin his portions were but didn't say anything until I went to pay. He explained that the cake was so rich that most people had trouble finishing even the smaller size. My work colleague laughed and told him that I'd have no worries whatsoever, so after reiterating how rich and filling the mud cake was, he immediately set me a challenge.

The deal was that if I ate two pieces of mud cake right there and then in front of him, he'd give me the rest of the cake free. Well I can still see the look of disbelief on his face when I polished them off in a very short space of time. It's not really something to brag about, but I was very popular in the office when I returned with enough mud cake for both morning and afternoon tea for everyone!

Some of my earliest memories involve chocolate. I can remember doing an experiment with my brother to see how little milk you could get away with in a glass spooned full to the brim with yummy Milo.

One of the treats about going to the movies is the candy bar food. I'd often polish off popcorn with extra butter, choc-top ice-creams and Maltesers or Jaffas, which I never wasted rolling down the aisles.

In fact, the only chocolate I detest is dark chocolate, it's far too bitter for me.

Researchers have now discovered what receptors eating chocolate releases in the brain that seems to have some sort of calming effect on me. But the more I ate, the more I wanted.

I knew I couldn't just have a row or two of that family block of chocolate and put the rest aside for later. I would keep coming back to it until it was finished. I could control it for a short time but then

I'd pig out again. Chocolate had a control over me and I wanted to be the one in control. I had to break the cycle.

There was no other choice but to put chocolate on my abstinence list and initially give up eating it altogether.

For the first few years I couldn't even have chocolate in my home. If ever I were given it as a gift I would always give it away immediately. I then became stronger and more confident that I didn't need chocolate to make me happy and found I could keep it in my fridge for visitors and not be tempted in any way to indulge, even in my darkest hour.

After about fifteen years of no chocolate I thought I was ready to go the next step and have a small amount, but my addiction was much stronger than my steadfastness and once I'd had that taste again my chocolate addiction was back and out of control once more. Chocolate's been the hardest component of my food fuel to control and once again I've had to totally abstain as I can't manage to eat it in moderation.

## Sweet tooth

I always knew I had a sweet tooth but it became very apparent when I first discovered the delicious taste of Krispy Kreme doughnuts. I had heard glowing reports about them but the first time I'd actually had one melt in my mouth was after a live *Beauty and the Beast* club show at Penrith Panthers. Next door was the first store in Australia and the length of the queues of people and the traffic lined up at drive-through staggered me.

Stan Zemanek and beauties Carlotta, Belinda Green, Jan Murray and me along with our crew, arrived in a minibus and as we were leaving, Panthers' entertainment manager at the time, John Hansen, presented us with a few dozen doughnuts to enjoy on the homeward trip.

The assorted filled ones were yummy but the glazed doughnuts were to die for. They were still warm so they just melted in the mouth and I was immediately hooked. They are as light and fluffy as fairy floss and I needed three to feel like I'd had the equivalent of one traditional doughnut. From memory Stan and our driver were the only ones on the bus who didn't overindulge and sample too many of them on the ride home.

Not long after that, Chris, one of crew at TVSN, started to bring them into work occasionally and I had to resist eating them. When I brought a couple of dozen in to reciprocate, I had to put them in the boot of the car so I wasn't tempted to eat them on the drive back.

I actually overdosed on Krispy Kremes when I was staying overnight in the hotel alongside Penrith Panthers. I went out to support Shannan Taylor at the boxing and discovered how tempting it was to have this enormous Krispy Kreme doughnut store open 24 hours a day 7 days a week.

As I wandered back to my room after the event I found my legs taking me across the car park and into the store where I bought some glazed doughnuts. They weren't hot but the attendant informed me that if I put them in the microwave for eight seconds they would be like new again and she was right.

I didn't have a microwave in my room so the doughnuts I devoured before going to bed and for breakfast the next morning weren't nearly as delicious as the ones I microwaved when I got home. And again, I had to put those in the boot or they wouldn't have lasted the long drive home into the city.

As they were rotating around the carousel of the microwave I began to read the box and was stunned to see there are 12 grams of fat and 7 teaspoons of sugar in each doughnut – for the glazed and the assorted crème ones just escalate up from there to around 22 grams of fat and 8 teaspoons of sugar. I vowed after this discovery that I would never buy them again.

Maybe I should have promised myself not to eat them again. I was helping out the Spastic Centre (now Cerebral Palsy Alliance) promoting their Cerebral Palsy (CP) Awareness Week and the first event was doing live weather crosses with Grant Denyer on the Seven Network's *Sunrise* program. One of the sponsors of CP Week is Krispy Kreme doughnuts and it wasn't long before dozens of these warm, mouth-watering morsels arrived.

It was a very early start and a little too early for me to stomach any food before I'd left home. I came armed with some fruit and I had already resisted all the cakes and biscuits that were laid out for everyone to enjoy. But the smell of the warm doughnuts was too much and I promptly ate one, then two, then three. That was almost my entire day's fat allowance and three days' sugar allowance gone just for breakfast! There were tens of dozens being handed around and without blinking an eye I could have easily eaten another three, but at least stopped myself and didn't do any more damage.

I was proud that same afternoon when, still as part of CP Week, I played in the celebrity team against some of the Australian Paralympic soccer team players, all of whom have cerebral palsy, which, by the way, didn't stop them thrashing us 7–3.

At the end of the game the Krispy Kremes were in plentiful supply, not only didn't I eat any this time around, but I'm sure the exercise from playing in the soccer match would have gone at least a small part of the way towards balancing out the damage I'd done earlier with the doughnuts.

## Choosing unleaded foods

Fat has more than twice as many calories/kilojoules as protein and carbohydrates. It's amazing how much your tastebuds change without you realising it. For instance I have been drinking skim milk for so long, if I do ever accidentally have full-cream milk it tastes like cream and is far too rich for my palate now. You might relate to how much you dislike the sweet taste after you've weaned yourself off putting sugar in your tea and coffee. You don't realise how much your tastebuds have changed until someone puts it in by mistake.

I have a big appetite and used to enjoy smothering a baked potato with lots of butter and sour cream and chives ... now I try and eat sweet potato and add plain yoghurt and chives instead. While I'll admit it doesn't taste the same as the sour cream, it does, nevertheless, taste really delicious and better than not having anything on the potato at all.

STILL HALF MY SIZE

Once again, I can't emphasise enough that you need to read the label on everything you buy and especially when it comes to low-fat foods. Many of them have exceptionally high sugar and salt levels, which are also vital to keep an eye on. Instead of snacking on potato chips (approximately 32.4 grams of fat per 100 grams) you might want to substitute pretzels (approximately 3 grams of fat per 100 grams) or rice crackers (approximately 0.9 grams of fat per 100 grams) instead. It's easy to pop your own corn but be careful not to put too much salt and butter on it. Better still, instead of consuming too many carbs and saturated fat in these snack foods, try eating a handful of nuts (not roasted or salted) that have heart healthy unleaded fats that will make you feel full.

## I'm now a veg-aquarian

Protein is a vital part of every cell in our body. It plays a major role in generating new cell growth, repairing cells, making antibodies to fight infections and is essential for new hormone growth and carrying oxygen in the blood. Some animal sources of protein can include milk and yoghurt, cheese, lean meats, chicken without the skin, fish, and eggs. Vegetable based proteins include tofu, nuts, beans and pulses, soy milk, rice and wholemeal bread.

After a lot of research and advice I once again altered my food fuel mix to incorporate lots of fish and seafood, on the proviso these foods are grilled or stir-fried and not battered or deep-fried.

## Pre-packaged foods

Out of all the weight-loss programs and fad diets that I ever tried, I've never tried pre-packaged foods but have known many people who have, all with varying degrees of success.

Being a big eater, I never found the portions big enough for me, but I watched a friend of mine shed almost 60 kilograms on pre-packaged foods. It took her about a year to shed all that body weight and she looked amazing. We were all as proud of her as she was of herself, but sadly when she stopped eating the pre-packaged foods and needed to start making her own decisions about what and how much she'd eat, drink and how much exercise she'd do, she slowly fell back into her original behaviours. My heart went out to her when she regained the original 60 kilos, plus another 10 kilos in less time than it took her to shed it all in the first place.

I've often wondered if it would be easy to stay my dream car size and shape if I had enough money to employ my own chefs to make me tasty healthy food and personal trainers at my beckon call. Then I think about a billionaire like Oprah Winfrey, who purportedly earns an unbelievable $90 million dollars a year and has chefs and trainers at her fingertip but she still has a constant struggle with her weight. There's a lot more to it than just putting good food into our mouths.

Oprah's trimmed down again and is looking stunning at the moment and looks like she might keep it off this time as she has literally put her money where her mouth is. Oprah attributes her success this time round to Weight Watchers and has become such a fan that she's bought 10 per cent of the company. Shares in Weight Watchers more than doubled when the news broke making Oprah around a $45 million paper profit.

## Breakfast

I don't think I have read any weight loss or health book that doesn't tell you that breakfast is the most important meal of the day and despite all this advice, for years I just couldn't stomach anything first thing in the morning.

The word breakfast literally means to break fast and is really important to kick-start our metabolism after it's been resting overnight while sleeping, otherwise you'll trigger the famine response I described earlier. Now studies prove that eating breakfast also improves your mind, your memory and your mood.

If you miss breakfast you'll find that you are often starving by mid-morning and then it becomes much harder to muster the willpower to resist having a sweet biscuit or three or a fat and sugar-laden muffin with your morning cuppa.

One of the reasons I think I couldn't eat breakfast in the past was because I had eaten too much food the night before, and more than likely too late in the evening, so most of the time I simply wasn't hungry when I woke up. I continue to find it hard to tolerate food really early in the morning but these days I eat less per sitting and try not to eat too late in the evening so that I wake up hungry instead.

We've all used the 'not enough time in the morning' excuse to miss brekkie and I'm sure it's been justified most of the time. There are a few tricks to help you squeeze in a bit of breakfast in whatever limited time you might have in the mornings.

Check the day before that you have all the ingredients. While it's all part of the discipline of getting up early enough to give you the time for what you need to do, if you're in a big rush in the morning or don't have a clear head when you wake up, you could perhaps save some time and set everything up the night before, ready to go.

A smoothie is a quick and easy breakfast to make. In a blender I put skim milk, half a banana (or use any fresh or frozen fruit you like), a raw egg, vanilla bean paste and lots of ice and blend it until it's like a thickshake. I've also substituted the milk with very juicy peeled oranges and blend them together with a raw egg (for protein) and ice. Both versions taste delicious.

Another quick breakfast for me to prepare is a bowl of fresh fruit, yoghurt and a couple of tablespoons of LSA (which is Linseed, Sunflower Seeds and Almonds). You can buy LSA already blended in a packet from your local supermarket but I think it tastes like chaff. It's easy to make it yourself and it tastes yummy. I've always been advised to keep the linseeds in the fridge as well as the LSA once it's made because once you break open the linseed (also known as flaxseed) it starts oxidising and if it's pre-blended in a packet stored on the supermarket shelf it will lose a lot of its goodness.

The LSA formula is three parts linseed, two parts sunflower seeds to one part almonds. I use the small blending cup of my magic bullet and blend each seed or nut separately but not too much so they don't go powdery, and then mix them all together.

If you add a couple of tablespoons of LSA to your fruit smoothie when blending it will add some great crunchy texture and delicious flavour and the fat and protein from the nuts and seeds will make you feel fuller for longer.

Have you ever read the label on yoghurts? Or compared brands? It's alarming how much sugar is added to yoghurt. I discuss the hidden sugars in food with Pete Evans and Dr Gary Fettke at the end of this chapter and Dr Gary includes a link to lots more information, including the added sugar in yoghurt.

## Shiftwork and your body clock

When I first worked with Clive Robertson at Channel 7 in the late 1980s and again at Radio 2GB through the 1990s he would always lament the terrible effect shiftwork had on his sleeping and eating patterns. While I was sympathetic to his plight, I couldn't fully appreciate what Clive was saying until I'd experienced years of shiftwork for myself and I must say Clive had just cause to complain as my body clock doesn't like it one bit.

The worst was doing midnight to dawn talkback shifts on 2GB. My first was in 1994 and my last was in 2016. Not only was it unnatural for me to stay awake throughout the night but I had to be mentally on the ball as well.

I would come off-air at 6 am all wound up and try to wind down and sleep when I got home. The whole time I worked through the night I never felt quite right during the day. That permanent ill feeling meant I definitely didn't feel like exercising and would tend to favour stodgy foods to buffer the unnatural changes that shiftwork was putting on my health and wellbeing.

Another shiftworking stint, again on radio, was when I filled in for Kayley Harris whenever she went on maternity leave when she was co-hosting WS-FM breakfast with Hans Torv. I found this marginally easier to cope with, as I could at least go to bed at the right time, even if it was an early start. WS-FM was in Seven Hills back then and as often as I could each day after coming off-air at 9 am, I would don my exercise gear and go for a big long walk with

Rebecca Orr, who was part of the Brekkie team, up and down all the hills around the studio that gave the suburb its name. I knew that if I didn't exercise then I would get too tired as the day progressed and end up not doing any exercise at all.

When I returned to live in Sydney again in 2010 I found myself back doing midnight to dawn on talkback radio on 2GB, 4BC, 2CC and some regional stations on the Macquarie radio network. I was hosting my own show on the weekends and would occasionally do fill-in for Brian Wilshire or Mike McLaren through the week.

I panelled the show myself, which meant I was responsible for the program going to air smoothly, or not – for all the correct commercials to be loaded and played during the entire shift, to come on and off delay and to cross to the news at the precise time. While all this was happening I also had to field talkback callers, keep up with breaking news, conduct interviews and competitions and try to keep my listeners entertained.

It's hard work and you really need to concentrate. I found working midnight to dawn left me feeling jetlagged for the rest of the week and threw my eating patterns entirely out of whack. The impact on my health was once again horrendous.

My heart goes out to every shiftworker reading this book, especially our first responders; our police force, ambulance and hospital staff who work rotating shifts, which I would find an absolute nightmare.

Dave Gorr and the late Phebe Irwin were an extremely successful award-winning breakfast radio duo on Wave FM in Wollongong and had to get up before the birds to entertain their listeners each weekday. You can read my interview with them about the effects of permanent shift-work on their health and fitness in Chapter 7 'Secrets from the stars'.

## Make a list and shop on a full stomach

There is no doubt that when I go grocery shopping I am more inclined to buy healthier food if I shop on a full stomach.

Making a list and not deviating from it is another helpful tip I learnt from attending weekly Weight Watchers' meetings. If you follow this guideline you're less tempted to weaken your resolve. And you might find that you'll spend a lot less money by not impulse buying.

## Water

I'm sure I don't have to sing all the praises of water and how important it is to drink lots of it, and regularly. I'm very lucky that I actually enjoy the taste of water and I don't find it hard to drink my quota of at least eight glasses of water a day.

I meet a lot of people who don't drink enough water. In fact, the comment I hear the most is they simply don't remember to drink it.

Anna, a mate of mine, who I regularly power-walked with in Wollongong, would lose count of how many glasses of water she was drinking per day but she knew it wasn't enough. She needed prompting so her simple method was to leave a big glass on the sink at home to remind her to have more water when she was at home. She also purchased an inexpensive child's postcard-size blackboard that she kept on the kitchen sink with some chalk. Each time she downed a glass of water she'd chalk it up and soon found she was keeping up her daily quota.

If you're struggling to drink enough water, try to have a glass or two when you first wake up. A squirt of lemon juice in it is ideal. Have another one when making breakfast and be sure to sip even more if you take vitamins and minerals.

If you make yourself a tea or coffee for morning tea try and get into the habit of having another glass of water while the kettle's boiling. And always make sure you drink lots of water when you exercise.

Having a big glass of water before you eat your meals will give you a fuller feeling in your stomach and I find it tends to stop me from overeating. But I have a bad habit of drinking a lot of water while I'm eating, which I believe is not ideal if you want to get the most nutrients out of the foods you eat.

There are times when I get water-logged and find that I need to occasionally put something in the water like a little bit of fresh lemon juice just to change the taste and ensure that I'm still keeping my fluids up. I don't drink tea or coffee so occasionally when I want a hot drink I'll have boiled water or add a small amount of lemon juice to boiled water.

# Pete Evans interview

Pete Evans is an award-winning internationally-renowned chef, restaurateur, published author, television presenter and a judge on Channel 7's *My Kitchen Rules* – the highest rating TV series in Australia.

Pete's hosted many TV shows that centred on travel, food and cooking, he prepared a royal banquet for Crown Prince Fredrick and our Crown Princess Mary of Denmark and he's showcased Aussie produce at the gala G'day USA dinner for 600 in New York City. His Hugo restaurant was awarded the much lauded chef's hat eight times and they won best pizza in the world.

Many chefs use lots of salt and butter to make food taste delicious but Pete is very passionate about embracing a happier and healthier lifestyle and the cornerstone to that is using food as medicine.

I met Pete Evans in the green room at Channel 7 in Sydney in 2015 when I was a regular on *The Morning Show* with Larry and Kylie and he was there to show how to make a fabulous paleo dessert on camera.

Not only is Pete 'drop dead' gorgeous, he exudes this amazing effervescent energy and he couldn't have been kinder or friendlier. I was carrying far too much weight at the time and lamented as much to Pete as we were chatting about the sugar-free dessert he was making and he shared a few interesting new findings about sugar that caught my attention and then kindly offered to show me his program, 'The Paleo Way'.

No long after meeting Pete, I was approached by *New Idea* to be hypnotised to see what difference, if any, that could make to shedding the kilos and keeping them off. I was both excited and nervous about being hypnotised but jumped at the opportunity and I'll explain that journey in more detail later in Chapter 5 'How do I say NO and mean it?'.

When I started reading up about 'The Paleo Way', my first thought was that if I could stick to it, then it would prove that the hypnosis was working, but in fact the reverse happened.

When I stopped eating refined sugars, bad fats and refined carbohydrates like pasta and bread, my sugar cravings disappeared.

It also created a positive domino effect on me; including calibrating my tastebuds to once again appreciate just how sweet whole fruit and vegetables do taste, finding I'm not as hungry so I'm not eating as much, I'm feeling and being more energetic and as a visual reward: a reduction in my size and shape.

In fact, the lifestyle eating plan that Tim Thornton, the hypnotist, gave me to follow was along similar lines to Dr Gary Fettke's LCHF Low Carbs Healthy Fats and Pete's 'The Paleo Way'.

**Susie:** Pete, you've been around food all your life and you're a certified health coach with qualifications from the Institute for Integrative Nutrition. What are the key issues causing Australia to be in the top five most obese nations on Earth, with over half of Aussie adults and a quarter of their children now overweight or obese?

**Pete Evans:** Hi Susie, I strongly believe it comes down to the fact that we as a society are so disconnected from nature and not only where our food comes from, but also from our own self-love. Once you love yourself completely, then you will make the wisest of choices to nourish your own body and of course your children. Nourishing your own body is one of the highest forms of self-love, whereas poisoning your body with alcohol and poor food choices demonstrates that you want to punish yourself for something. This opens up many different pathways for one to explore how best to make the wisest choices in regards to self-love.

**Susie:** What is the basis of your documentary *The Magic Pill*?

**Pete Evans:** Our film *The Magic Pill* showcases the power of using real food as one of the tools to health along with modern medicine ... we need the best of ancient wisdom, coupled with the best of modern science.

**Susie:** Is there any sugar that is okay to eat in moderation?

**Pete Evans:** I don't think sugar is an evil thing, I just think we need to understand blood sugars first and foremost and then work out how much carbs we really need for health, which is why a low-carb approach is the most sensible.

**Susie:** What about alternatives like honey or stevia?

**Pete Evans:** As above, a little honey or stevia or organic sugar is not evil, but if you are eating carbs in excess of what your body needs then each gram of carb or sugar if you like, is going to add to your health problems.

**Susie:** Wouldn't school canteens be the perfect place to start educating our youth about good nutrition and begin by banning soft drinks and junk food and providing more healthy alternatives? Surely, these foods, highly laden with fat, sugar and salt, are contributing enormously and adversely to our ever growing childhood obesity crisis?

**Pete Evans:** Ideally every parent would make their children lunch at home so the children can take it to school. You cannot shift responsibly as a parent to a school canteen.

**Susie:** How can we dispel the myth that eating supposedly 'diet' low-fat versions of certain foods like yoghurt is a better alternative, when in many cases, the fat taken out is replaced with harmful levels of sugar instead?

**Pete Evans:** We should be getting off dairy first and foremost as dairy from a cow has only ever been created for a young cow for a small period of time. As for low fat, that myth is well and truly dead for anyone with eyes to read the latest nutritional science or to join social media pages that promote healthy fat.

**Susie:** What are the best ways to curb our sugar cravings?

**Pete Evans:** Start eating a 100 per cent low-carb paleo approach and include fermented veg and bone broth. Once you start eating this way, you will not only stop craving sugar after about six to eight weeks but you will probably only feel like eating two meals a day!

**Susie:** I'm not sure why some of your peers are trying to silence you but please explain 'The Paleo Way' eating principles and why you feel it is the best food fuel mix for us to run our body at its optimum?

**Pete Evans:** 'The Paleo Way' is about eating the most nutrient dense and nourishing foods on the planet for our species – humans. We have evolved being hunter and gatherers (omnivores) so we eat animal fat and protein as well as plant-based foods – not one or the other but both! By eating this way we nourish our body and give it the fuel that it loves. An abundance of colourful vegetables, a moderate amount of well-sourced seafood and or land-based animals (the fattier the better) and if you can eat nose to tail even better (organs, bone broths, cheaper cuts) then enough healthy fat to satiate either from the animals or you can use eggs, nuts, seeds, olives, avocado, coconut etcetera. Add some fermented veg and bone broth for good gut health and make sure each meal looks like the above … simple.

**Susie:** What made you decide to adopt 'The Paleo Way'?

**Pete Evans:** I needed to love myself and make the most of this life.

**Susie:** What changes, did you notice when you started living and eating 'The Paleo Way'?

**Pete Evans:** I have become better on all levels – health, mental clarity, you name it, it has improved and continues to improve.

**Susie:** Why isn't dairy part of 'The Paleo Way'?

**Pete Evans:** Because every mammal drinks its own mothers milk (or species milk) for a period of time then is weaned onto once again its species' own specific diet. For instance, a baby cow is born and drinks its mother's milk (if it is lucky these days) then after a period of time moves onto grass, which intuitively it knows is its food. No animal returns for more milk past its adolescence when it becomes mature, so why on earth would humans go from our perfect food as a baby (our mother's breast milk) and think that a cow or goat is better for us, or even entertain the thought of consuming milk after weaning. Add to this the ethical nature of how most dairy cattle are treated and what they are fed and then what happens to the milk and you don't need to be a rocket scientist to understand that this is truly not a health food for humans. If you don't believe me, then give it up 100 per cent for six months completely and see how you feel then reintroduce it.

**Susie:** It's very hard to get true healthy alternatives when you eat out, especially at lunch time, where you might only have time or access to fast food and food courts. Any suggestions on what the best food options are for us to choose?

**Pete Evans:** When you eat paleo 100 per cent low carb then you will probably only eat two meals a day (I generally eat one to two) so lunch won't be a problem if you have eaten breakfast and you want to skip it, if you don't have any existing health issues. If you believe you have to eat then stick with vegies and meat/seafood/eggs. Simple

**Susie:** What's the single most important thing you feel we need to do to make a positive change to our health?

**Pete Evans:** LOVE OURSELVES.

# Dr Gary Fettke interview

Dr Gary Fettke is a very busy orthopaedic surgeon from Launceston, Tasmania who has authored *Inversion: One Man's Answer for World Peace and Global Health*, which is now available free online.

Dr Gary launched and mentored Nutrition for Life, a diabetes and health research centre based in Launceston. His website Nofructose.com is gaining momentum and respect globally.

I was introduced to Dr Gary by Pete Evans and was so appreciative, as were my midnight-to-dawn talkback listeners, when Dr Gary agreed on numerous occasions to give up his sleep, take talkback calls live on-air and discuss his passionate mission to reverse diabetes with his LCHF Low Carbs Healthy Fats food fuel mix.

Live on radio Dr Gary openly shared his own battle with obesity as a child and the weight related issues affecting his patients' joints and arthritis. These were the catalysts for his longstanding interest in preventative health outcomes, and particularly before operating on his patients. Dr Gary's also a cancer survivor and an environmentalist.

**Susie:** What is sugar also labelled as in pre-packaged foods?

**Dr Gary Fettke:** Sugar is labelled in more than 50 different ways. Labelling identifies ingredients by type and many pre-packaged foods have more than one type of sugar and can confuse people, particularly if listed in what appears to be a random order. (www.healthline.com/nutrition/56-different-names-for-sugar#section9)

**Susie:** Is there a difference between added sugar and sugar that comes naturally from whole fruits and vegetables that we eat?

**Dr Gary Fettke:** Sugar is sugar. It is just glucose and fructose. Fruit tends to have a higher amount than vegetables. On the whole vegetables have minimal sugar and generally have more vitamins, minerals, fibre and phytonutrients than fruit. A small amount of seasonal and local fruit is part of living to your environment. Many non-seasonal and imported fruits have been treated in a variety of methods which can decrease their nutrient value.

Frozen berries lose a lot of their nutrient value after three months of storage.

**Susie:** Why can drinking fruit juice and fruit juice concentrate be as damaging to our health as drinking soft drink? Why are 'diet' soft drinks also bad for us?

**Dr Gary Fettke:** Whole seasonal fruit comes with fibre. That can slow up the body's absorption of the sugar. It does not change the overall load. When fruit (and vegetable) is juiced and/or concentrated the fibre is broken down and the sugar is absorbed rapidly requiring the secretion of insulin by the pancreas. This is the same effect as drinking 'soft' drinks (as we have been marketed the term 'soft' drinks).

Diet soft drinks can be just as harmful. They do not generally have as much or any sugar in them. The sweeteners still drive some recognition 'sweetness' pathways which are associated with eating behaviours, obesity and type 2 diabetes onset. There is a varied literature on the chemical side effects of artificial sweeteners. Avoiding them is a good start even before consideration of potential chemical effects.

**Susie:** Is there any sugar that is okay to eat in moderation?

**Dr Gary Fettke:** Sugar is sugar, again. We have been marketed this term 'in moderation'. My take on it is that if I have sugar, added or natural, it tends to make me hungry for some hours, lethargic and tired after that and keeps me awake at night. Not dissimilar as the effects seen on children at parties where they indulge in more than 'moderate' sugar intake.

I am satisfied with the WHO recommendations of trying to keep added sugar to less than 5 per cent of total calories. No added sugars for children under two years, less than four teaspoons of added sugar for children and about six for adults. I personally aim for no added sugars apart from that found in fresh 'real' food.

**Susie:** What about honey or a sugar sweetener like stevia as an alternative?

**Dr Gary Fettke:** Honey is still fructose and glucose but the percentages vary with type. It will have the same effect as table sugar. The added advertised 'natural' benefits are really quite small. Remember that when we eat honey we are taking it away from bees that rely on it for their winter hibernation. It's a careful balancing act for beekeepers. Harvesting honey from wild beehives is potentially devastating for those bees.

Stevia is a 'natural' sweetener and we presume it is safe but it has not been studied as extensively as other sweetener agents. Many people find it quite 'metallic' in taste which puts them off. My concern is that you are still reinforcing that 'sweet hit' when eating food. That has potential problems like those found with artificial sweeteners. We don't know enough yet.

**Susie:** What do you class as polyunsaturated seed oils?

**Dr Gary Fettke:** All oils and fats that we eat are a combination of saturated, monounsaturated and polyunsaturated oils. The percentages vary and the ratios of omega-3 to 6 vary. We need a certain amount of polyunsaturated oils but the amount has increased greatly on the last few decades and particularly the percentage of omega-6 oils, which tend to be more inflammatory, based on their ability to be oxidised. The seed and vegetable oils have a few names and are higher in percentage of polyunsaturated oil. Common names include canola oil, vegetable oil, soybean oil, sunflower oil, cottonseed oil, margarines and butter-spread substitutes.

**Susie:** What are the best fats and oils to eat instead?

**Dr Gary Fettke:** I don't recommend masses of fat and oil. We tend to cook with butter and well sourced olive oil. Coconut oil and lard have low percentages of polyunsaturated oils. Avocados and fish have an excellent profile too.

**Susie:** I understand that all disease starts from inflammation. Why does eating sugar and polyunsaturated fats make them such a lethal combination that can harm our good health?

**Dr Gary Fettke:** The consumption of sugar and polyunsaturated seed oils combine in our diet to create inflammation in every blood vessel wall and in every tissue in every organ of the body. The addition of refined carbohydrates including bread, white rice and pasta only aggravates the damage process. Fructose

(50 per cent of sugar), polyunsaturated oils and refined carbohydrates look to be the major contributors to most of our modern conditions including obesity, diabetes, heart disease, dementia, cancer and a raft of other conditions. This is the problem for us all and our children … right now!

**Susie:** How important is it to eat local and seasonal produce?

**Dr Gary Fettke:** Fresh food that is local and seasonal is by definition, Low Carb Healthy Fat living. Real food does not have much sugar and carbohydrate in it. Refining and milling practices are actually processing whole grains, so I recommend avoiding them and getting your 'fuel' from pasture-raised animals, healthy fats – and that includes dairy if you are not lactose intolerant.

**Susie:** I'm not sure why some of your peers are trying to silence you but please explain your LCHF Low Carbs Healthy Fats eating principles and why you feel it is the best food fuel mix for us to run our body at its optimum?

**Dr Gary Fettke:** It's not my medical peers that want to silence me. The 'anonymous' complaints have stemmed from dietitians that believe in the old paradigm. The trouble is their textbooks have been saying the same thing for decades. That social experiment of cereal and grain-based advice, anti-meat and anti-full fat has turned out to be a total health and economic disaster. It's time to rethink.

**Susie:** Wouldn't school canteens be the perfect place to start educating our youth about good nutrition by banning soft drinks and junk food and providing more healthy alternatives? Surely, these foods highly laden with unhealthy fat and sugar and salt are contributing enormously and adversely to our ever-growing childhood obesity crisis?

**Dr Gary Fettke:** School canteens would be a great space to start but there is resistance because of the dollars. Real fresh food takes time to prepare and store carefully. That equals less profitability and more staff. The long-term cost needs to be considered both in health and academic results but that is beyond the average school environment. We could start serving decent breakfasts and lunches (cost included in education) and improve learning whilst at school. (See the following website for the French lunch model: karenlebillon.com/french-school-lunch-menus/)

**Susie:** How can we dispel the myth that eating supposedly 'diet' low-fat versions of certain foods such as yoghurt is a better alternative, when in many cases; the fat taken out is replaced with harmful levels of sugar instead?

**Dr Gary Fettke:** Back to that education. The visuals are the way to go. I love the comparison video of how much sugar is in yoghurt, highlighted in this skit on the ABC's *The Checkout*: (youtu.be/ HUPMAlNHBiU)

**Susie:** What's the best way to curb our sugar cravings?

**Dr Gary Fettke:** Two ways. By avoiding sugar, you will avoid the hunger as long as you replace the sugar with essential proteins and some healthy fats. Then listen to your body. Don't eat by habit. Eat when you are hungry and keep the portion sizes down. Most people are amazed how the hunger goes when the sugar and carbs reduce.

Don't let others undermine you. When they try to do that it is often their insecurity that you are doing what they actually want to do but have not tried. Lead by example. You might just surprise yourself.

Don't see it as a failure if it takes a while for the cravings to go. It's 'only' a lifetime of sweet hits that you are trying to overcome. Cutting back is a great start.

**Susie:** As an orthopaedic surgeon, what does carrying extra weight do to our joints and the rest of our body?

**Dr Gary Fettke:** Carrying too much weight is not just harmful to joints, it also hurts more. Obesity and inflammation increase joint disease, and there are the risks of surgery associated with treating them. Changing to healthier choices means many people can actually avoid surgery completely. Why not seriously try it?

**Susie:** I remember you telling me on talkback radio that when you started as an orthopaedic surgeon, you might have done one amputation every six to twelve months and now they are happening weekly. What's causing this increase in patients requiring surgery?

**Dr Gary Fettke:** My public hospital practice in northern Tasmania has a lot of people with the complications of diabetes. Those complications can be completely avoided with an avoidance of sugar and reducing carbohydrate significantly. For many it's too late and we are having to do debridements of feet every week with far too many new patients. It's so sad for them, their families and the community.

**Susie:** You were part of a fascinating experiment on Channel 7's *Sunday Night* program, where three people, with diabetes were each put on a different eating plan. One was placed on 800 calories a day, one ate carbs and fruit and Tony from Tasmania made the lifestyle changes to embrace your LCHF Low Carbs Healthy Fats regime. What were the results? How did Tony go?

**Dr Gary Fettke:** Tony did fabulously over the twelve-week intervention. He lost, I think, about 15 kilograms, lost his arthritic knee pain, came off five medications and brought his blood tests down to non-diabetes levels. He is a year down the track now and delighted to still be lighter and healthier, and still off those medications.

**Susie:** Can we reverse this type 2 diabetes tsunami by just eating the right food and of course education?

**Dr Gary Fettke:** Yes. The complications of type 1 and type 2 diabetes are completely avoidable with a low carbohydrate lifestyle.

**Susie:** Most of us are aware of type 1 and type 2 diabetes but I think you'll shock those reading this book when you explain type 3 diabetes.

**Dr Gary Fettke:** The term type 3 diabetes is being applied to early onset dementia. It is a flow-on effect of poorly controlled diabetes. It is devastating families and particularly our Indigenous communities. The tragedy is that it is completely avoidable with a low carbohydrate healthy fat (normal protein) LCHF lifestyle.

**Susie:** What's the single most important thing you feel we need to do to make a positive change to our health?

**Dr Gary Fettke:** For me, it was understanding that our cells require essential proteins and healthy fats to fuel ourselves. There is no absolute requirement for us to eat sugar and carbohydrates. Our body can make them from other sources. In nature, sugar and carbohydrates are seasonally available and we, as animals, tend to eat them at the time of plenty to make us fat for the lean winters. The trouble is the sugar is there every day and there are no 'lean' winters any more.

## Susie sums up

- Visualise your body as your dream car

- Choose the best fuel mix to suit you

- It's natural to crave fat – just eat more unleaded than leaded fats

- Monitor your high- and low-octane carbohydrates

- Don't forget to eat protein

- Eat breakfast

- Anything in moderation or abstain until you can

- Go grocery shopping on a full stomach

- Don't be a martyr – treat yourself

- Drink plenty of water regularly

# Weight-loss tips from celebrity lips

**Trevor Hendy:** You need to be healthy in your mind, believe in yourself, be happy with yourself. So if your life is a certain way then your weight is probably reflective of your state of mind. So start by looking at how you feel about things and ask 'What do I do the same every day, what is the pattern? What is not working for me?' And if it's going to upset people around you to change that then gently, gently change it. If you really need to change it fully then let them deal with it in their way.

**Dave Gorr:** Everyone says drink water but I hate water, I absolutely hate it and I get up in the morning and I make myself drink half a litre of water first thing out of bed and then it's done. That's all the water I'll drink probably for the day. Even though I know I should be drinking at least three times that much, I can't drink it. If someone could invent water that didn't taste like water, maybe like cordial, which I think there is but I don't think it's as good for you as water is.

**Phebe Irwin:** My tip would be don't fool yourself; every single thing that goes over your lips counts. It just adds up. It does.

**Sandra Sully:** Portions are the key. Most people don't realise their portions are creeping up in size. When I was growing up a steak was a third of the plate and vegies were two thirds, but have you noticed how much that has changed? A steak is now two thirds of the plate and vegies are a third. The concept of the appropriate portion for a meal is completely lost so people are eating too much in one hit and the wrong quantities of the wrong things.

**Fran Macpherson:** Exercise, exercise and more exercise. You know the greatest thing about exercise is when you are doing it you feel thin.

**Jeff Fenech:** Watch what you eat. Eat healthy and exercise. It's no use being 55 kilograms and not being able to walk down the street, so you've got to exercise as well as eat right. If you have a night where you eat or drink too much, have a routine in place to work it off over the next day or two.

**Shelley Taylor-Smith:** Everything in moderation, even moderation. If you want that Tim Tam, have the Tim Tam. Treat yourself: you deserve it. Be good to yourself because you deserve it. You're the best, forget the rest. It's one of my mottos. It's not a good emotion to feel starved, so treat yourself, because you are a gift.

**Jessica Rowe:** Balance. Balance things, don't think, 'Oh my God I'm depriving myself.' Eat mainly healthy, but don't feel too guilty if you splurge every now and then.

# CHAPTER 4

# GET YOUR MOTOR RUNNING

The title of this chapter and the first few lines of the Steppenwolf song 'Born to Be Wild' illustrate the cornerstone for adopting a philosophy to permanently maintain your dream car at its optimum shape and performance level. Getting the correct mix of food fuel is only one of the things that will allow your dream car to stay on the road to success. Another is to ensure that you regularly clock up some kilometres on your body's odometer. Exercise is paramount and works best in unison with monitoring your fuel consumption.

## How much fuel can I burn?

You'll find a chart on the Mayo Clinic's website with the amount of calories you can burn in one hour doing 32 different exercises and activities. If you work in kilojoules then multiply the calories on the chart by four.

The three columns show three different weights in pounds 160 pounds equals 72.5 kilograms, 200 pounds is 90 kilograms and 240 pounds equates to around 109 kilos.

According to the Mayo Clinic 3500 calories (14,000 kilojoules) equals 1 pound (0.45 kilograms) of fat. If we exercise and burn 500 calories (2000 kilojoules) a day or eat 500 calories (2000 kilojoules) less a day we will lose 1 pound (0.45 kilograms) a week on average.

The result will be even better if you reduce your food intact and increase your exercise at the same time and don't forget to compare some of those Mayo Clinic exercises with Dr Rosie's chart at the end of Chapter 11 'Add sex and double your results'.

## Anything I can do, you can do better

Thinking about it, I can never remember my parents ever playing any sport or doing any exercise outside of physical daily work. While they were rarely idle, their activities would generally be work-related or involve completing chores. If Mum and Dad relaxed, it would be to rest or socialise, never to exercise, except on the rare social occasions they'd dance cheek to cheek. As a chubby, awkward child I found it was easy to follow in their footsteps.

You might be reading this and thinking that you're not really cut out for exercise either but take heart that you won't ever be as hopeless at it as me. I'm not exaggerating. When it comes to sport and exercise, anything I can do, you can do far better. Just touching my toes has always been and still is a challenge for me. I've never had a very good sense of balance. My knock-knees and fear of heights only compounded the fact that sport was never really my forte. As a young child, despite pillows strapped to my waist and backside to cushion the blows, I still couldn't keep upright during my innumerable attempts to learn to roller-skate up and down the hallway of our home.

At school, sport was compulsory and as keen as I was to participate, to be frank, I really wasn't good at any sport I tried and there were certain things that I was actually pretty bad at doing. Jumping hurdles is one that immediately springs to mind. I was often the laughing-stock of everyone on the sideline as I managed to knock down every single hurdle during athletics and then had to go back and help set them up again for the next race.

My lack of sporting prowess didn't stop there. In team sports I was always the weakest link and never expected to be picked for any competitive side. More often than not I held the position in every team of Left Right Out.

We could choose our sport in senior high school and as boys were high on my curriculum, in winter I chose ice-skating. There used to be an ice-skating rink at Narrabeen, on Sydney's northern beaches, which was only one suburb away from our school. A couple of schoolmates and I would think we were so cool because we didn't have to wear our sports or school uniforms and we were trying to make a good impression with the boys.

Often my optimism far outweighs my genuine capabilities. In this case, despite visualising myself effortlessly gliding across the ice, Torvill and Dean style, I found myself in the same predicament I'd faced years before during my disastrous attempts at roller-skating, but this time I was minus the pillows. I ended up looking most uncool, spending much of the time either clinging white-knuckled to the rails or trying to pick myself up after landing on my bum on the wet ice.

Even Mum, who always tried to be positive and supportive, used to smile and simply say, 'Oh well Susie, you can't be good at everything, at least you tried.' I never seemed to be good at anything to do with sport and always felt bad about letting the side down.

There is a great deal of evidence now that all points to how exercise not only keeps your chassis looking sleek but it is also great for keeping what's under the bonnet in peak condition as well. Exercise improves your state of mind as it releases feel-good endorphins in your brain. It also improves your circulation and so many things related to your general good health.

## What exercise is best?

One of the best exercises I've found to help reduce my size and shape is to regularly push myself away from the dinner table. You'll find great fitness tips from my contributors at the end of this chapter. What was clearly reinforced to me while I was doing the interviews was that it doesn't matter what sort of exercise you do; just make sure you enjoy doing it and you continue to do it.

It's very important for our body engine not to be just idling all the time. We have to take it out of first gear and hit the highway to burn a bit of fuel and clear out the carburettor. That'll help to keep our engine running at its best and enable us to unhitch the box trailer we feel we're carrying around our rear end sometimes.

Exercise can also prevent a lot of injury. As I get older I can only hope that increased blood flow is also helping to keep my important internal body parts functioning at their best, giving me a longer, healthier journey through life.

Just like our motor cars, we all need to service our body vehicle on a regular basis. If you've been 'up on blocks' on the couch for a while or only venture around the block occasionally, please go to your GP for a check-up before you embark on any exercise program. Like a good qualified mechanic, your doctor can give you a professional check-up, service, grease and oil change and the green light to venture on whatever journey you have in mind to burn your food fuel intake and change your shape to resemble your dream car, while making it the smoothest ride.

Pain is your dream car's dashboard warning light telling you that something might not be functioning at optimum level either physically or emotionally and the pain can often pinpoint the part of your body that is out of kilter. Don't let the problem compound and then find that your local GP has to send you off to a specialist to fix it.

Unfortunately it's not as easy to get replacement parts and fit them in your dream car body, as it is to an automobile you drive around in. It can get expensive and a major repair may require you to be put in hospital overnight or for a few days, all because you ignored your pain's warning light and left it too late for a simpler fix-up from your local GP.

By the same token, don't confuse pain with muscle soreness that you get through exercise, especially when you start up again after a long spell. Stretching before and after exercise and massaging the muscles can minimise the soreness.

You might not have a problem with overeating but often it's the exercise part that lets you down. It's so easy to find an excuse not to exercise. It's either too hot or too cold, you're too busy, can't get a babysitter, there are security issues, ill-health or cost; whatever the reason, another day passes and still no exercise. And it doesn't help if you've got a sedentary job, perched in front of a desk or computer all day.

I now have a variety of exercises that I enjoy and that I can incorporate into my busy lifestyle.

## Gym classes

Over the years I've tried many gym classes, and embraced new techniques such as step classes and pump classes but I don't think aerobic workouts are for me. I find it too jarring to pound my body through a routine on a gym floor.

A stunning woman who is no stranger to television is journalist and news anchor Sandra Sully, best known for hosting Network Ten's *Late News* nationally and prime time *News at Five* in New South Wales.

One of Sandra's little-known talents is that she is a qualified fitness instructor and you can read more about her qualifications and achievements along with an insight as to how she stays the size and shape she is, in Sandra's interview in Chapter 7 'Secrets from the stars'.

## Walking

Most of the 50 plus kilograms of body fat that I'd shed and written about in my first book *Half My Size,* along with all the other kilos I've shed since, have primarily been through walking. It's easy, it's free and no matter how flat your tyres feel, you can start to pump them up a little bit by beginning, literally, with baby steps and taking long flat walks before building up to incorporate some hills and stairs.

In 1991 when I was recovering from glandular fever, I couldn't do anything but walk and that was excruciatingly slow and exhausting to begin with. After spending ten months flat on my back and despite everyone telling me that you lose stacks of weight when you have glandular fever, not surprisingly, I put on heaps of weight instead and my fitness and motivational levels were at an all-time low. At first I barely had enough energy to walk to my front door, it took months before I could go from my apartment block to the end of the street and back. It was through perseverance and determination that I was able to slowly do a bit more and a bit more. Until finally I was able to power walk about 8 kilometres return, up the beach from North Wollongong to Towradgi and back.

One of the great things about walking is you can do it anytime and anywhere. It can be most enjoyable if you have a companion or a pet, or if you're in a group. But it's also something that, more often than not, I also enjoy doing on my own. I listen to the radio with headphones and depending on the time of day and my mood I either listen to music or talkback radio. Occupying my mind while my feet are pounding the pavement makes the time fly past.

Now I have mapped out a few walks of varying lengths and intensity around Glebe and Pyrmont in Sydney's inner west and the walk I tackle depends on the time I have to spare. By wearing my heart-rate monitor (I've detailed what it does and how you measure your heart rate later in this chapter), I'm able to see at a glance if I'm still training in my fat-burning zone and how much my heart rate increases when I go up a flight of stairs or a steep hill and how quickly it drops on the straight stretches.

## Wrist weights

Unless it's on a sandy beach at the water's edge I've never enjoyed running. It always leaves me very red in the face, often with a headache and sore breasts. I found after walking for a few years that my fitness level had increased to a point where my heart rate no longer reached its fat-burning level when I was swiftly walking on flat ground and swinging my arms. Running wasn't an option and if I wanted to keep walking then I had to find another way to increase my heart rate overall. I wanted the hills and stairs to spike my heart rate and put it into a higher cardiovascular level but still be in my fat-burning zone on flat ground so I purchased a pair of strap-on wrist weights. These weights are only one kilogram each, which doesn't sound very heavy, but by simply swinging my hands with these attached to my wrists, I find I can increase my heart rate immediately. Over a longer time I've noticed they have also helped to tone up my arms, back and breasts.

I see many people carrying hand weights when they're out walking but I prefer having my hands free. I'd also find it too uncomfortable to keep my hands clenched all the time holding onto these weights. My wrist weights are firmly strapped to my wrists with Velcro. This allows me to swing my arms freely while I'm walking and to do a series of toning exercises and pump my hands to move the build-up of fluid back through my body without putting any strain on the joints or muscles.

## What exercise equipment should I buy?

There is no doubt that you need a combination of good eating habits and exercise. Over the eight and a half years working on *Good Morning Australia (GMA)* I was often asked to recommend exercise equipment. My answer would always be the same – whichever one you are going to use all the time. Too often these pieces of home gym equipment become expensive clotheshorses or you end up buying a year's gym membership in good faith and only go once or twice. No prizes for guessing why most of the exercise equipment you see at garage sales looks like its brand new.

## Heart-rate monitor

One of the best investments I've ever made is my heart-rate monitor. Nikki Anderson, a fantastic freelance make-up artist/ hairdresser and former head of hair and make-up at Channel 10, used to do my make-up most weeks for *GMA*. We used to chat about losing weight and exercising and her wealth of knowledge seemed endless. Nikki's always kept fit and her husband at the time owned a series of exercise equipment stores. Nikki was the one who explained how beneficial a heart rate monitor would be for me and she was spot on.

I started seeing quicker weight-loss results when I started using a heart-rate monitor and would you believe it's not because I wasn't working hard enough. Quite the contrary, it's because I was working too hard. Yes, I was working in my upper cardiovascular range, which is very good for your health, your fitness level, heart and blood flow, but it's burning mainly sugars rather than stored fat.

To work off the stored fat, she explained that I need to work at around 65 to 70 per cent of my maximum target heart rate for 40 minutes or more, and to push myself into my upper cardiovascular level for short bursts during this time to increase my fitness level and burn more kilojoules.

## How do I calculate my maximum target heart rate?

It's easy … 220 minus your age. So if you are 30 years of age then your maximum target heart rate is 220 – 30 = 190 beats per minute. And 65–70 per cent of that is around 120+ beats per minute.

If you're not in a position to get a heart rate monitor or fitness watch or you don't have access to a heart rate monitor app on your mobile tablet, then you can check your pulse manually by placing your fingers (not your thumb) on your jugular vein or wrist and time your pulse over ten seconds – remember to count zero on the first beat – then multiply it by six to calculate your heart rate per minute.

## Incidental walking

I first heard this term at the Golden Door Health Retreat, located in the hinterland of the Gold Coast. As Golden Door is built on the side of a mountain, there was a considerable amount of incidental walking just going up or down from my cabin to the dining room, pampering rooms or the swimming pools and back.

It is possible to incorporate quite a lot of extra exercise into your day without even being aware of it. As an example, if I have to drive somewhere and I have the time, I'll try and park my car at the opposite end of a street and walk up and back rather than park close by. I'll also try and take the stairs instead of the lift as my first preference. My apartment building has a lift but I'll opt to take the 82 steps from my car park to my front door whenever I can.

## Dancing

My first introduction to dancing was when I was in early primary school. Our fabulous neighbours at the time used to include me in a lot of their activities. One of their daughters, Julie, who is incredibly talented in music and dance, was going to classes at Harbord every Saturday morning.

I started in the beginners' class in tap and modern jazz. It gave me a good sense of rhythm but I was so much bigger than the other kids in my class and nowhere near as graceful or coordinated. We had an end of year concert that combined a lot of the classes to perform together and I'll never forget one of the routines, which was to the music of the *Pink Panther*.

We were all dressed up as panthers, Julie was the star performer in pink out the front and the rest of us were black panthers. I was the big chubby kid in the back row. In hindsight, I probably looked more like I was doing the baby elephant walk than the Pink Panther, but I enjoyed myself nevertheless.

In the 1980s I really enjoyed attending Jazzercise classes, as they were choreographed exercise routines set to the latest music currently playing on the radio and you could sing along to the songs while completing the routines. In the early 2000s I did some salsa and Latin dancing classes and a belly-dancing course and I believe that dancing is one of the most underrated forms of exercise.

Dancing has been best described as 'the vertical demonstration of the horizontal desire'. You'll be amazed at how fast your heart rate increases when you dance, vertically or horizontally.

If you'd like to know more about how many kilojoules you actually burn during 'horizontal folk dancing' and how it stacks up to other activities then check out Dr Rosie King's graph in the unsealed section in Chapter 11 'Add sex and double your results'.

## Boxing

Nothing has toned my body or changed my shape more than boxing. My first introduction to boxing was in 2001 through one of my dear friends, dazzling television presenter Sami Lukis. Sami enlisted me as her boxing partner down at the Police Boys Club at Woolloomooloo and she sets a very high standard.

I'd already met Jeff Fenech and his gorgeous wife Suzee a few times at a number of charity functions and learnt firsthand the incredible generosity of Jeff and Suzee. Jeff always made himself available for interviews and was one of my 'blokes' in a fun segment called 'Susie and the Blokes' that ran regularly during my afternoon talk back program on Radio 2GB. It was a popular segment best described as a reverse radio deviation of the television show *Beauty and the Beast,* where I was 'the beast' asking listeners' questions to my panel of blokes. Since then I've had the chance to get to know and adore the entire Fenech family.

I readily accepted Jeff's kind invitation to train me at his gym between his professional boxers. Who wouldn't jump at the chance to be trained by a three times world-boxing champion? Not me, that's for sure.

I was excited and nervous at the same time. I didn't know what to expect and more importantly if I'd be able to cut it. The first day I arrived at the gym I expected it to be abuzz with boxers and trainers stretching, sparring and working out, but they all started arriving after we had already started training and everyone was very friendly.

Jeff had me warm up for ten minutes on one of the bikes while I strapped up my wrists. Then on went the boxing gloves and we got straight into the ring. Jeff used hand pads and instructed me to punch into them in different sequences, correcting me all the time.

When I first started I barely lasted 30 seconds before needing about a minute to recover. I was already in a lather of sweat and wondered how I would ever be able to last a full three-minute round. Jeff was very encouraging and didn't push me too hard. I knew that the more I trained, the longer I would able to last and the quicker I would be able to recover. I had a clear goal to work towards. Before I knew it, I could spar with Jeff for the entire three-minute round, with a 30-second break in between. And at my fittest Jeff had me doing 8 x 3 minute rounds with 30 second breaks in-between and often joked that I was fit enough to do amateur boxing. Jeff's the best trainer I've ever worked with as he never let me overdo it, however, when he felt I'd improved he would increase and vary my work-out and then started me lifting weights.

Jeff may have hung up the gloves on his own professional boxing career but he's still passing on his wealth of knowledge and experience to his Team Fenech boxers and is heavily involved in training and promoting up-and-coming boxers. Jeff Fenech shares his story and some fantastic fitness and motivational tips in his interview in Chapter 7 'Secrets from the stars'.

## Golf

It was George Bernard Shaw who described golf as a good walk spoilt by a little white ball, but I have to disagree entirely with him on that one. I wasn't introduced to the joys of golf until I was in my early forties, prior to that I'd only had a bit of a 'hit and a giggle' at corporate and charity golf days. If I'm ever asked if I can play golf, I often respond that my nickname's 'Lightning' and not because I'm fast or straight down the line but more aptly because I never strike twice in the same spot. It generally gets a laugh and covers me for those extra 'practice shots'.

Eventually I discovered that I have the perfect temperament for golf. It's an ideal game for me because I'm the only person I ever have to beat and I never let anyone else down in the process. One hole at a time is the way I approach golf and I don't care if I botch it up as there's always the next one.

With the number of shots it takes me to play long holes, I end up getting more golf for my money than most people. I'm lucky that I can generally hit them fairly straight down the fairway although I have been known to give out a Homer Simpson sounding 'Doh!' from time to time.

## Yoga

Not only don't I have a very good sense of balance but I'm also not very flexible and have never been able to touch my toes, which my very first chiropractor assured me was not necessary anyway. As comforting as that might be now, I've always envied girls who can do the splits and bend over and put their hands behind their knees and touch their knees with their nose.

My first yoga experience was in Wollongong in the mid-1970s and I think that turned me off going for almost 30 years. I felt so out of my depth and uncoordinated that I could never imagine being flexible enough to enjoy the class. I can best liken it to taking the two years of violin lessons that I struggled with in high school and expecting to play with the Sydney Symphony Orchestra today.

The class was run by the most talented, tiny Indian woman, who was so flexible I thought only contortionists could get into those positions. Yoga classes were rare then but this class was packed. The teacher was revered by her peers and had been featured in magazine and newspaper articles alongside other famous yoga names such as Roma Blair, who had a yoga show on television at the time. I was in my early twenties and the teacher only looked like she was about ten or fifteen years older than me, but she was certainly extolling the virtues of yoga when she announced that she was actually in her sixties.

This yoga teacher was so patient and I persisted a few times but eventually gave up. I found it all too slow and I never managed to drift into that meditating state that kept everyone else so still for so long at the end of each lesson.

Yoga didn't become the buzz word in exercise until the late 1990s and since then its popularity has spread like wildfire. Suddenly magazines and newspapers were featuring articles and columns dedicated to the practice. They also started quoting all the celebrities who favoured yoga and what type they were doing. I was contacted by the producer of *Yoga TV* and asked if I'd do a segment with one of the hosts, Kylie Jaye. I welcomed the opportunity to learn more and found Kylie to be extremely passionate about yoga and with an ability to explain things so well that even someone like me could understand.

I hope everyone watching found it amusing to see me attempting to replicate some of the positions that Kylie could easily weave her way into. Kylie has such a vibrant personality and an inward calm at the same time. She explained that yoga is an holistic approach of the mind, body and soul. Even after the cameras stopped rolling Kylie generously continued to give me her tips on food as well as exercise.

But it wasn't until 2002 that I ventured back into a yoga class and that was thanks to the incredibly effervescent Janie Larmour from The Centre of Yoga.

Janie Larmour has been in the fitness industry since 1994, firstly as a personal fitness trainer and then yoga instructor. Her clients have included some of the 'who's who' of the film, fashion, music and magazine world.

I first met Janie during a 'Chardy Friday' segment on the marvellously talented Cleo Glyde's afternoon show on thebasement. com, a live web-based music show originally established by the legendary Doug Mulray. During the live telecast Janie showed us how she easily earns the nickname 'The Human Pretzel' by putting both her feet behind her ears and rocking like a turtle on its back. The show was flooded with emails from around the world from internet viewers praising Janie's abilities and asking her all sorts of questions about yoga and fitness.

Janie was a welcomed guest on the Nine Network's *Fresh* program and for two years made many new fans as a regular on my national daily variety and lifestyle show *SUSIE,* where she displayed many times to my Australia-wide audience via the WIN Network and Channel 9 in Perth and Adelaide, her expansive yoga knowledge along with her ability to turn into a 'Human Pretzel'.

Janie's graced the cover of *Australian Yoga Journal,* regularly contributes to magazines and websites and spends much of her time teaching and training yoga students globally online, alongside running her Sydney yoga studio. Janie's regularly invited to travel overseas to contribute to yoga conferences and conduct yoga workshops where she showcases her Zen Ki Yoga to an international audience.

I've drawn on her vast experience in the fitness industry and her down-to-earth approach to health, fitness and weight loss, to guide us through the plethora of different yoga styles and classes.

According to Janie, there are no rules with yoga. All styles work and not one of them will harm you as long as you work within your abilities and limits. She says that if you're wondering which yoga is the best one for you, it comes down to personal preference. The most important thing is to try each one until you find one you like. Also, be aware that you will need to find a teacher (or teachers) that you like as many students have given up yoga because the teacher was intimidating or pushed them too far, too quickly.

Janie Larmour helps explain the different types of yoga below:

### Hatha

This is the most common form of Indian-style yoga and literally means 'force' or 'effort' in Sanskrit. While it may be gentle, it can also be strong, depending on the student's level of ability and the actual style that is applied within the class. Hatha can be used to describe the actual type of yoga and is also a term used to describe many other different styles of yoga (for example, Iyengar, Astanga, Vinyasa etcetera can all be considered to be Hatha yoga).

### Hot yoga

This was originally called Bikram yoga but due to the founder's legal issues, many studios have changed the name. The room is heated up to 37° C and for 90 minutes you do a series of 26 poses in sequential order. Some studios offering Hot yoga have varied the sequence. The room is heated to the body's natural temperature and is thought to decrease injuries as the muscles are warmed.

## Iyengar

Iyengar can be stronger than Hatha; postures usually involve a lot of set-up with equipment to ensure safety. It can be slower and postures are held for longer as the muscles and breath are more deeply focused on.

## Astanga

Astanga (sometimes spelled Ashtanga) is a very dynamic form of yoga where the student progresses through each series of sequences, which builds on the previous one. Astanga is a yoga that keeps you constantly moving and definitely builds your strength as well as your flexibility.

## Power yoga

This is a practice also done in a heated room, but usually a little cooler than Hot yoga, around 30° C. The sequences are well-rounded to cover all parts of the body. The practice can be challenging and great fun.

## Viniyoga

In Viniyoga, students are taught that the breath should actually lead the body into and out of each posture to create an awareness of how the yoga affects the individual and the practice is adapted to find the balanced and appropriate postures for each person.

## Vinyasa yoga

Again, different styles of yoga can be called Vinyasa yoga such as Astanga, Power or anything that has a rapid flow of sun salutations synchronised with the breath. Vinyasa flow is another popular term that you may hear.

## Kundalini

Kundalini energy is normally described as a sleeping or coiled serpent, which is located at the base of the spine. All yoga will tap into this energy to some degree, but Kundalini yoga concentrates on it specifically by using its power and safely guiding it.

## Zen Ki yoga

While there are several forms of Japanese yoga based on zen shiatsu, the five seasons of oriental medicine and a macrobiotic diet, I have refined these styles and combined it all with modern exercise science and good old common sense to pioneer my own style, which is Zen Ki yoga.

Aside from it being a total mind-body system, it tones muscles and organs and works the energy meridians just like acupuncture and shiatsu as well as keeping you flexible and supple. Zen Ki yoga has become an incredible healing system for alignment problems that may be causing pain and other health issues.

There are specific poses to help strengthen the bladder, your intestines, help with serious digestive issues, women's health issues and modern mental health issues such as anxiety, panic attacks and much more.

You can find more information about Janie Larmour's The Centre of Yoga on her website, where she has an enormous variety of yoga DVDs and training sessions available to suit beginners through to those who also want to become a yoga teacher: www.thecentreofyoga.com.

According to Janie, a great way to lose weight is to simply chew your food. That's it. Chew your food. Yogis say you should chew each mouthful 150 times before swallowing but even Janie admits that she's never been able to achieve that! But she says that when you chew your food properly you are breaking down every bit so that your body can use it. The chewing action creates saliva in your mouth so the more you chew, the more saliva you are creating in your system, which will fill your belly and therefore you need less volume of food to fill you up.

# Glenn Chipperfield interview

As each year passes, not only does it appear to fly by quicker than the last, we also seem to have less and less time for ourselves to do the fundamental things to keep our dream car in tip-top shape and healthy under the bonnet.

Exercise is one of those 'must do's' and despite all our best intentions, when we start hitting the potholes in our life's journey, more often than not it's exercise that gets sidelined for a variety of reasons.

As we age it's very easy to become less active, especially if we start feeling some aches and pains, which is why we need to choose new ways to maintain our health by venturing into more suitable regimes that include diet and being active.

Just like going to a mechanic to service your car, we need to visit our health and fitness professionals to keep our motor running smoothly.

Glenn Chipperfield has been playing an active role in the fitness industry since 1972. Glenn's a registered teacher and has spent almost two decades as a TAFE course coordinator and head vocational teacher and more recently delivering adult education and training including diploma courses in fitness, business and management, sports management and sports development.

Glenn's the Australian inventor, designer and creator of his 'fitness centre in the water', the world renowned Aqua Bladez, he co-founded ten Healthworks Fitness Centres and is a much sought after corporate mentor.

In amongst all of Glenn's vast experience and qualifications, Glenn's also skilled as a fitness trainer for children and older adults and in addition to him sharing some of his best fitness advice in this chapter, you'll find his quick and easy exercises the family can do in the TV commercial breaks, without venturing too far from the couch listed in the back of this book.

**Susie:** What are some of the flow on effects carrying extra weight has on our body?

**Glenn:** Carrying extra weight impacts on our entire body, as well as the known concerns of diabetes and heart disease, the excess weight may cause issues with our joints.

If we consider movement patterns for those of us carrying excess weight in our thighs, with them rubbing together we tend to take wider steps, which alters our natural movement patterns and can cause issues with our body alignment. If we observe people walking who are holding weight around their mid-section we may notice their arm movements tend to swing across and around the body thus causing a swaying action at the hips. Instead of lifting our knees when we walk, carrying extra weight can cause us to throw our legs out changing our walking action, which can have negative impact on weight-bearing joints.

An article from Harvard Medical School stated[*] 'When you walk across level ground, the force on your knees is the equivalent of 1½ times your body weight. That means a 200-pound (90 kilogram) man will put 300 pounds (136 kilograms) of pressure on his knees with each step.'

Each time our foot strikes the ground pressure is transferred through our joints. To ensure this pressure is distributed as evenly as possible our body needs to be in alignment allowing the bones and joints to move in the most natural ways they were intended. Landing with our feet further apart may cause soreness in the ankles or knees. Running increases the pressure as we touch the ground and excess weight can cause soreness in our main weight-bearing joints. Therefore wearing appropriately fitted, good-quality footwear can be beneficial to help minimise the damage on these joints. To follow on from your car analogy; if the wheels aren't aligned then your tyres will wear down differently. The same goes with your body.

Check the soles of your shoes to see if there's an even or uneven pattern of wear. Is there more heel wear on one leg or one side? Is the outside worn down more? You may be favouring one leg or hip and this may cause lower-back pain.

---

[*] Why weight matters when it comes to joint pain. Harvard Health Publications, 2015

www.health.harvard.edu/pain/why-weight-matters-when-it-comes-to-joint-pain

STILL HALF MY SIZE

Get a friend to video you from behind whilst you're walking along (but it needs to be when you're unaware for it to be as natural as possible) and only for about six steps. Replay and watch your movement and see if it looks natural and balanced. We look at ourselves in the mirror all the time and come to grips with our appearance but the view from behind will allow you to decide if you may need a consultation with a relevant health professional.

Carrying extra weight has a flow on effect on our spine too. A physiotherapist recently explained to me that an extra 1 kilogram around the waist can create 3 kilograms of excess strain on your spine.

We hear the term core muscles and these refer to the muscles around the mid-section of our body that assists in keeping us upright. If these are neglected this may cause an imbalance and create pain in the lower back. The strengthening and maintenance of these front and rear muscles is important. Try strapping on a loaded backpack in reverse so the weight is hanging in front of your stomach. You'll immediately feel the strain on your lower back as you try to stay upright. This will give you an idea of what you're expecting your back to tolerate every day to support you if you carry weight in the tummy region.

**Susie:** There are so many simple lifestyle influences that regularly impact on our posture, what's your best advice to right these wrongs?

**Glenn:** Correct posture works to minimise the impact of gravity, however, we develop poor postural habits from bad seating positions, when we're hunched over a computer or using other technology, pushing prams, trolleys and strollers and even when driving a car. As a result unnecessary strain can develop, our shoulders become rounded and a forward-tilting head causes tension in the upper spine. When our body gets out of alignment, our muscles need to work harder to keep us upright and that's when pain and injury can start to develop. We also need to acknowledge how much time we have our head tilted forward whilst on our phones, computers and other electronic devices. All these actions cause us to use more of our chest muscles than our back muscles and all this is exacerbated when we're carrying extra kilograms.

To begin remedying this process, a simple antidote is to stand tall and imagine you're holding a grape between your shoulder blades. As you take a deep breath imagine you're crushing the grape by squeezing your shoulder blades together and hold briefly. Aim to repeat this at least ten times throughout the day, particularly after sitting or typing on a computer for an extended period.

**Susie:** Not only are most of us time-poor but we want instant gratification. There are no short-cuts to getting into shape are there?

**Glenn:** It's actually really important not to rush it. Start out slowly then gradually increase the intensity, instead of overdoing it and risking injury or giving up because it's all too hard. It may have taken us years to be where we are so let's start the journey with a plan and one step.

A simple 20-minute walk (10 minutes out and back) is a great way to begin and listening to music or the radio at the same time keeps your mind distracted. Use music that makes you want to move. As you get fitter you can increase the intensity in spurts by walking quicker between two driveways or two power poles then go back to walking at your usual pace and gradually try to repeat these higher intensity bursts of energy more frequently as your fitness improves. Start incorporating some stairs and hills/inclines into your walk as you start to feel better and stronger.

I worry about those TV weight loss reality shows where they fast-track morbidly obese contestants into doing excessive amounts of exercise, while drastically reducing their food intake. Not only don't they have a great success rate of contestants keeping their weight off after the winner is announced and the cameras stop rolling, I'm actually more concerned at the ongoing damage this extreme training is having on the contestants. Also, giving viewers the perception of large weight loss in a short time period is not realistic.

**Susie:** What are the possible implications of carrying more weight than our bodies were designed to carry?

**Glenn:** Your car has a recommended towing and carrying weight. If it is exceeded it may have a negative impact on performance and possibly damage some parts of the car. Likewise, when we carry excessive weight, over time our physical performance starts to diminish and our body may begin to develop and suffer health issues.

If a car is parked and not being used, it can develop problems over time, usually beginning with a flat battery, the tyres may go flat and parts will need lubricating. If left standing idle for too long your car can seize up. Your body will also start changing and developing unhealthy complications if you don't keep it moving. Not only is there a possible weight gain but a lack of strength and muscle wastage; a good example is how atrophied an arm muscle gets after being placed in a plaster cast for six weeks. Medical experts are suggesting sitting is the new smoking. By doing regular exercises that you enjoy you'll actually gain more energy, improve your mental health and help you get your dream car shape and size.

**Susie:** What made you invent your Aqua Bladez?

**Glenn:** I have been an aqua fitness instructor for over 40 years. Regardless of your age, water is the perfect place to exercise. Besides being pleasant and relaxing there is minimal compression of your joints. Aqua Bladez allows a backyard swimming pool or any safe body of water to become your own private gym. I've designed Aqua Bladez with progressive strength training principles in mind. You simply glide them through the water in various directions and at different speeds using the water as resistance. As you slowly increase the resistance and repetitions, you'll start building muscle, improve your level of fitness, strengthen your core muscles, improve coordination and balance, assist in weight loss and help avoid the weight-loss plateau. It's also a fun way for children to exercise and help fight childhood obesity. The rehabilitative exercises I have designed for the Aqua

Bladez are intended to challenge and strengthen your body and help you fight the ageing process for as long as possible.

Instead of going to the fridge or the cupboard to get more food during the commercial breaks, Glenn Chipperfield wants you to utilise the time and try his quick and simple exercises that can easily be done on the couch or in front of the TV to stay active and begin the process of adaptation and habit formation. Glenn says to create habits that we enjoy we need to experience small successes or gains along the way. The mistake fitness instructors often make is thinking pain is always good. Athletes can understand this process but for most people pain means 'not fun'. If we do things that are good for us and progress slowly from one to two to three etcetera we can count the gains and see long-term results.

Check out the Glenn's exercises in the back of this book and involve the whole family and have fun doing them together and seeing who can do the most or who can bend the deepest.

# Susie's simple steps for getting into shape

- Regularly burn your food fuel intake

- Find an activity or activities you enjoy

- Stick with it!

- Take baby steps

- Monitor your heart rate

- Get the green light from your doctor to start

- Keep challenging yourself to do more

- Incorporate exercise into your daily routine

- Where possible take the stairs not the lift

- Park your car and walk

- No matter what activity you choose be sure to move your body!

# Fitness tips from celebrity lips

**Wayne Pearce:** My best fitness tip is to do something on a regular basis. Doesn't have to be intense, as long as it's regular, even walk on a regular basis, three or four times a week, that's a great start.

**Tara Moss:** My best fitness tip is to be happy. Because if you are a happy and content person you'll do the right amount of exercise to stay that way. I think fitness is a lot of different things. You have got to find what works for you. What makes you happy, what keeps you at your optimum level? And that to me is fitness. If you're in tune with your body you will start to do the things that will make you feel better. That's why I think excessive exercise can be as harmful as no exercise. I believe it is about a balance.

**Fran Macpherson:** I think you have to work it out for yourself. For me, it's running, walking, dancing and sex.

**Jeff Fenech:** My best fitness tip is to enjoy what you are doing. Don't go and do something because you think you should, or don't do something you don't like. Unless you're happy you never give your best, you never feel your best afterwards. So be happy and enjoy what you are doing, I think it's the tip to life in general.

**Shelley Taylor-Smith:** Consistency. If you don't quit you'll make it; that's my motto in life. No matter where you are in your life, it's always the right time to start. There's no wrong time. Wherever you are, the hardest step is the first step and once you have taken the first step, you are on your way to success and the new you!

**John Maclean:** Have a balanced program, as it is with most things in life. Start off and gradually build up. Muscles adapt to stimuli so if you increase the exercise gradually you'll find that you get stronger, physically and emotionally from it.

**Jessica Rowe:** Work out what's right for you. Don't be pressured into following a fad or thinking I've got to be doing this because this is the trendy thing to do or so-and-so is saying I must do it.

Follow what's right for you, listen to your own heart, trust yourself.

**Trevor Hendy:** My best fitness tip is if you're being true to yourself and you're walking that path and for a week or two you haven't found the time to exercise, it's okay. Probably the number one tip is not to push. Don't force yourself in a way that takes you out of the zone where you are being true to yourself.

# CHAPTER 5

# HOW DO I SAY NO & MEAN IT?

'Minds are like parachutes, they only function when open.'
- THOMAS DEWAR

My mind can be the biggest handbrake that stops me from cruising along my road to success with the top down on my dream car with the wind in my hair. Willpower, or rather the lack of it, has been one of my biggest stumbling blocks to achieving my aims and goals. Why is it that this emotional strength sometimes eludes us despite all our best conscious thoughts and intentions? And then why do we feel guilty and punish ourselves when we don't live up to our inner expectations? Do we set far too high a standard for ourselves, that we can't ever be expected to attain?

## Self-esteem

What is self-esteem? I checked the *Concise Oxford Dictionary's* definition:

> **self n.** *person or things own individuality or essence, person or thing as object of introspection or reflexive action*
>
> **esteem n.** *favourable opinion, regard, respect*

So basically it's what we think of ourselves, is it not? Well if that's the case, why is it so important to us what other people think and say and do? And why do we let it impact on us so much?

A female friend said to me recently, 'If you don't love yourself, how can you expect anyone else to love you?'

While that sounds great in theory, it's a hard thing to do at the best of times, let alone when there's self-doubt. So why does being stood-up, or cheated on, or passed over for a promotion, or not getting the job at all suddenly undermine our confidence, plummet our self-esteem and take us on an emotional roller-coaster ride, often with self-defeating results? Like, in my case overeating.

I think we're all realistic enough to know that we're never going to stop these glitches in life from occurring, but it's how we react to them that's important. For a balanced person, with strong self-esteem, these reactions are appropriate and proportionate.

I used to blame and hate myself and then revert back into the comfort zone that garaged my negative behaviours. Now I try and overcome the pitfalls so I can 'pick myself up, dust myself off and start all over again' instead of wallowing in my own self-pity.

A few winters ago I got a verbal 'slap across the face' from a male friend, whom I hadn't seen for a while. He said, 'Gee you've beefed up, I didn't recognise you walking down the street.' In fact, I'd put on a good dress size or two. While it might not seem much when you compare it to the 50-plus kilograms or the six dress sizes that I'd been able to shed and kept off for so long, it still concerned me greatly nonetheless.

To be honest, I had noticed my clothes getting tighter and how some things were getting much harder to do up, but they were simply relegated to the bottom of the washing basket. I didn't start to take any action to make anything fit me better until I felt my cheeks burning from his comments. I'm sure there was no malice intended but his words still stung at the time. In hindsight I was actually pleased he said it and it was definitely the catalyst that gave me the shift in paradigm I needed, to put me back on track … for a while at least.

Would you want someone to tell you you'd gain weight? Would it be too bitter a pill for you to swallow? Or would it make you go the other way and eat more? I wonder if I'd have taken as much notice as quickly if the comment had been sugar-coated or if it had come from another woman instead?

What do you think of yourself? A negative body image is one of the biggest contributors to low self-esteem. How often have superficial things like a pimple or a bad-hair day made you feel self-conscious? You imagine the pimple is standing out like an emergency beacon equipped with its own red flashing light and everyone is staring at it and you. You really want to hide under the doona all day but trowel on the concealer instead. And while make-up might have turned off the red flashing light, every time you look in the mirror, in your eyes, you still see the beacon. It then remains in the forefront of your mind and becomes quite a distraction. As a result your body language changes and you start to feel even more self-conscious.

Even though your uncomfortable behaviour might make some people think you're acting a little strange, the truth is, nobody really takes any notice of these minor imperfections. In fact, another friend believes you can't love something that is perfect. It's the imperfections in people that are endearing to us. Whether it's a temporary setback of an acne outburst or the more far-reaching results of family, peer group, media and social pressures; negative body images are formed over a lifetime of many different influences. So it may take some time and effort to change them, but it can be done.

What is this cultural tendency we have to judge people by their appearance? And why does it impact so much on our self-esteem? Why is it so important to us to be accepted by others? Why do we care so much about what other people think?

Sadly, many children who do the taunting at school were taunted themselves. They grow up and often continue the cycle as adults. If they have children of their own, invariably this inherent behaviour continues.

I was staggered to learn that Kids Help line, which provides an outstanding free, private and confidential counselling service for Australians aged between 5 and 25, receives thousands of calls per year from their youngest demographic, the 5–12 age group, with serious concerns about their body image.

Sometimes how you perceive and feel about your body may have no bearing on your actual appearance and it's not uncommon for women of Western nations to believe they are bigger than they really are. It's also estimated that about 45 per cent of Western men are unhappy with their bodies to some degree, compared with only 15 per cent some 25 years ago. Gay men and athletes are particularly vulnerable to poor body image or feeling insecure about their bodies.

'Your most important sale in life is to sell yourself to yourself.'
– MAXWELL MALTZ

So what do you think of you? You might not love yourself or even like yourself for that matter, but it's important that you believe in yourself and recognise and identify your best attributes and not just focus on the negative aspects about yourself.

I'll explain a simply way you can take a critical look at yourself in Chapter 10 'Smoke & mirrors'.

When you put yourself under the microscope and make your own personal blueprint, you'll be amazed at the number of things about yourself there are to list in your 'good points' column.

We do need to know both our pluses and our minuses, so we're aware of which bits we need to target and, where possible, attempt to improve our 'not so good points' list. But more importantly we need to take hold of all our positives and direct plenty of energy into highlighting them.

It's a good idea to re-examine your blueprint from time to time and when you do, be sure to reinforce and focus on what's positive about you and not just dwell on the negatives. You can use it as a springboard to measure your future success. If you don't want to write anything down then I'm sure you have a mental picture of what bits of yourself you're happy and unhappy about.

It's really important to get a good healthy balance. Many times when we embark on a new venture we tackle it full on and overdo it. I've had to learn to put things into perspective and not to sweat the small stuff because the older I get the more I realise … it's all small stuff!

# Willpower

In motoring terms, I guess willpower could equate to the bumper bars at the front and back of your car. Fortifying the chassis and the duco and helping to protect me if I hit any obstacles in my path. Or you might prefer to think of willpower as your shock absorbers, helping you glide over the rocky patches you hit along life's way.

Either way, both these features come standard on all dream cars; but each make and model varies so you'll need to find the correct switch that turns on your willpower and then learn to drive with it in action.

I admire internationally acclaimed comedian, actor and TV host Julia Morris for a lot of things: her wit, her talent and her friendship, but also for her incredible willpower.

We were both very big girls when she took me off in a skit on *Full Frontal* in the early 1990s and we became friends after meeting at the Logies and then often worked together on *Beauty and the Beast*. Not only have we shared the cover of *Who* magazine's 'Still Half Their Size' issue in August 2002 (see photo in picture gallery) but we've also shared many a delicious meal together after an exercise work-out on my regular sojourns to Melbourne. Julia's successful weight loss and maintenance has also been well documented, and Julia denies herself nothing. We both unquestionably admire each other's strong willpower, but I still maintain that Julia has far more willpower than I do and she feels the opposite.

You see, whenever we've gone out to dinner Julia always eats whatever she wants … but only ever half. If she has a hamburger and chips, she will cut and eat only half the burger and leave half the chips. That to me takes amazing self-control and as much as I'd like to think I had that inner strength, if the food was in front of me I know it would be torture for me, once I'd tasted it, to have to stop after only eating half. Then if I did only eat half, I'd have the biggest guilt trip about throwing away food while it was sitting in front of me. This mental tussle would ultimately result in me eating the lot, even though it would have been better in the waste than on my waist!

In 2004, Julia Morris was based in London and newly named *Time Out*'s Comic Of The Year, when we caught up for a yummy yum cha. Still looking trim, taut and terrific, I asked her how she still manages to find the willpower to leave half the food on her plate when she dines out. She did confess that on some occasions she had to squash her serviette into the plate to stop but had been known to lift the serviette and take just one more mouthful before completely wedging the serviette back on top of the leftovers. When Julia is eating at home she's very conscious of what she buys and tries not to bring unhealthy food into the house to tempt her and tries not to eat carbs after 2 pm.

The reason Julia thinks I have the stronger willpower is because I can totally eliminate certain foods like chocolate out of my fuel mix and she'd find that too torturous to deny herself something indefinitely. Julia's self-control wouldn't work for me and she wouldn't want to adopt my kind of self-restraint because the results would more likely end in failure for us both. We both have the same goal yet we have implemented totally different methods to exercise our strong willpower in slightly different ways. The key is to find what suits you.

If you're like me and don't think you could resist leaving half your food or only having a wafer-thin slice of your favourite cake, then I suggest you don't put your inner strength to the test. Maybe try avoiding it altogether until you think you can handle it and then treat yourself. No matter what we overindulge in, it's an obstacle course out there.

Every day I used to walk past the most divine French patisserie that was at the end of my street, and while I could always walk the long way home to bypass the cake shop, it's not so easy to avoid the ends of your fingers if you're a nail biter.

Half your luck if you don't have a problem with overindulging. But a lack of willpower might also be keeping us in an unhappy relationship or a job we hate or preventing us from saving the money for that much-wanted holiday or car.

I know there's much in all our childhoods that has contributed to our habitual actions, reactions and feelings, both positive and negative. How do we fight these impulses and gain self-control?

Can our conscious mind win out over our sub-conscious? The answer is a big YES: Julia and I are living proof.

There is no doubt you can succeed too if you are prepared to use your willpower. Celebrities share their willpower tips and ways to overcome obstacles at the end of this chapter.

## MMSOBGYTAST

Is resisting temptation really just putting it off until nobody is watching? My dear friend Geoff Sheehan encouraged me to spell out these eleven letters in magnetic scrabble pieces across the front of my fridge, level with my eyeline, so that each time I open my fridge I see M M S O B G Y T A S T.

It's short for: come 'mustard, mud, shit or blood grit your teeth and stay there!' This acronym and saying is taught to beginners learning formation flying in the RAAF – especially fighter pilots, for whom being in the correct formation may be a matter of life or death.

## Change

> 'Only a mediocre person is always at his best.'
> – SOMERSET MAUGHAM

No doubt we can all better ourselves in some aspect of our lives; and who wouldn't want to improve themselves physically, mentally, emotionally, spiritually, socially and financially?

It's always the things we don't like about ourselves that undermine our confidence and allow our low self-esteem to fester. It could be poor social skills or an emotional strain in our family life or a need to improve our health. Whatever the reason, nothing will change if we don't. And where there's no change, there's no improvement.

A few people including Albert Einstein and Mark Twain have been attributed as saying, 'The definition of insanity is doing something over and over again and expecting a different result.' Willpower requires change. So what's stopping us? Is it fear?

If so, is it a fear of failure? Or a fear of success? Unfortunately there are always difficult stages we have to go through with anything we want to change. If you've ever tried to do a simple thing like growing your hair, you'll know how easy it is to give up while you're going though that 'in-between' stage and get it cut off again.

I find abstinence is the only way for me to control some of my 'flairs for excess', but what works for me may not work for you. Finding what best suits me was very much a matter of trial and error, and I often learnt more from my mistakes.

In *The Seven Factors of Achievement,* author Pauline Douglas sets an interesting journal exercise and asks, 'If I dared to live a life that I truly loved – what changes would I make?'

## Be positive

B positive not only happens to be my blood group but also one of my most important mottos in life. I believe you can overcome just about any obstacle that you might encounter on life's rocky road with a positive approach and I'm not the only one who thinks like this. If ever I get the 'poor, poor pitiful me's' and think life's deck of cards has dealt me a rough hand, I think about swapping places with my nephew Matthew, who was born in 1988 three months premature and is severely disabled with cerebral palsy (CP) as a result.

It's estimated that a child is born with CP every fifteen hours in Australia, there's no known cure, no pre-birth test and the incidence and the severity of CP is on the increase. Mattie's breast plated into a wheelchair, and has a 270-degree curvature of his spine. He'll never be able to walk, has little to no control over any part of his body and while his speech is constantly improving, Matt's hard to understand at the best of times. He's blind in one eye and has about half a metre of extremely poor vision in the other resulting in Matt requiring 24/7 care for everything. Cerebral palsy is a permanent physical disability and there is an extremely sharp mind along with a wicked sense of humour trapped side Matt's twisted body.

Despite all of his disabilities and chronic pain, it's very rare not to see Matt without a huge smile on his face. I look at him sometimes and think if anyone has an excuse to bitch and moan it's him, but he doesn't (well very rarely). He's the only man in my life, who has ever shown me unconditional love. I'm so proud of him, as he has grown into a really great bloke and an incredible and constant inspiration to me.

Another person who has shown me how you can overcome huge obstacles to come back stronger mentally, physically, emotionally and spiritually is an extraordinary athlete and motivational speaker John Maclean. John shares his truly remarkable story in Chapter 7 'Secrets from the stars'.

## Depression and anxiety

I didn't realise that depression was a side effect of glandular fever and when this dark cloud started to descend on me again bringing with it anxiety attacks, overeating, low self-esteem, and feeling alone even in a group, I finally opened up about it to my GP Dr Jim during the weekly vitamin B12 shots he gave me to help improve my fatigue and boost my low concentration. And I'm so relieved that I did.

It wasn't the first time in my life that I'd experienced these symptoms but it was the first time I'd had it professionally diagnosed as depression. I've suffered bouts of it since during very stressful times in my personal and working life but I know what it is now and have sought lots of professional help to deal with it and try to overcome it.

'Did you overeat because you were depressed too?' was the first question Malcolm T Elliott asked me on Radio 2UE during an interview about my weight loss when I'd just made the front cover of *Who* magazine's 'Half Their Size' issue in January 2000 (photo in picture gallery). I'd never been asked that question on-air before but I knew Malcolm had battled his weight for most of his life and we ended up having a long discussion on the debilitating condition of depression.

Depression is not something you should necessarily try and battle on your own; there is so much help available now in so many forms. I prefer treatments that don't require taking medication. A very simple book called *Taming the Black Dog – A Guide to Overcoming Depression* helped me. It has been written and illustrated by the author of *Living With It,* Bev Aisbett, and is distributed to health professionals.

My glandular fever only started to clear up after I had my tonsils removed, which were constantly re-infecting my system, but the low self-esteem and depression didn't lift with it. Your mind can play terrible tricks on you, especially when you are in an enforced rest and can't do much else other than think.

One thing that did pull me out of my mental malaise to be positive again was getting a phone call from the blood bank. I've been a regular blood donor since I was eighteen but I hadn't been in to give blood or plasma since getting sick, which was close to a year. They were in urgent need of my rarer B+ blood type for a young boy with leukaemia. I told them of my illness and they checked and said it would be okay, so I immediately went and donated.

It might sound weird, but I felt better afterwards: more valuable and capable, maybe deep down it was because someone needed me. I had some self-worth back and from there I began to rebuild my health and my self-esteem. As hard as it was, getting back into exercise also helped dramatically. Not only in my fat reduction but also in lifting my depression by releasing endorphins: the 'feel good' hormones in our brain.

## Singing out loud

One of the best tips to control my anxiety came from a lovely doctor in Newtown. I was going through a really tough time mentally and I knew I had to seek medical help immediately. As Dr Jim is based in Wollongong and I live in Sydney's inner west, I rang up all the doctors' surgeries near me and was lucky one could see me almost immediately.

She was so helpful and understanding and when I dismissed the idea of controlling my anxiety attacks with prescription medication she suggested simply singing out loud. She went on to explain some of the recent studies she'd read about the correlation between singing out loud and lifting your mood and from personal experience the doctor was spot on. Now I often sing along to my favourite songs while I'm out walking.

## Control the urge to fall off the wagon – the four R's

Now when I'm feeling depressed, angry, sad or any of the other emotions that trigger my binge and comfort eating, I try and follow Dr Jim's four R's to fortify my willpower and stay on track. I don't always succeed but I no longer beat myself up over failures either:

**Relabel:** It's not me; it's my brain chemicals that are making me think like this.

**Re-attribute:** It's not me it's the stupid side of my brain.

**Refocus:** Think of something else, go off and do something else to distract and delay it by fifteen minutes.

**Revalue:** See how it is now, hopefully it is no longer important.

Dr Jim's four R's get a workout most often when I'm feeling low and crave very sweet or very fatty foods and I know I'm not really physically hungry. Now, instead of immediately giving in to these cravings, I firstly acknowledge that they are simply that – cravings. It's my brain not me.

Having assessed that I've had my quota and that I'm not really in any physical need for food, then I try and work out what's triggering these cravings. Something might be bothering me emotionally, or it might be hormonal, and whatever I identify it as, I relabel it.

If the cravings intensify instead of diminishing I re-attribute that it's not hunger and once again identify and relabel the problem then try and work out a solution. I then promise myself that I will not eat anything, especially the foods I crave, for at least fifteen minutes and refocus.

This generally means changing environments, if possible. For instance, if I'm writing at my computer I'll take a break and go and do a chore on my 'to do' list, or pamper myself with a quick facial, or put on my boxing gloves and do a few rounds on my punching bag or walk up the street and check my postbox. I try to do productive things that don't involve eating.

Then, more often than not, when I revalue those cravings they have disappeared and, in turn, I'm feeling good about myself for having the willpower to resist the unnecessary and unhealthy high-leaded and high-octane fuel that I had earlier longed for. If you do succumb to your cravings, don't beat yourself up over it and give up altogether because you've slipped up. Take a deep breath, put your brain in gear and Dr Jim's four R's in motion and start again.

It's worth reiterating that when I don't eat refined sugar or grains my sweet cravings disappear, immediately strengthening my willpower.

## Hypnosis

I've always watched hypnotists on TV with a great deal of scepticism, until I had four first-hand experiences, two of them on my national TV show *Susie*. The first was Leon W Cowen from the Academy of Applied Hypnosis, who took several of the production staff at WIN-TV and spent quite some time hypnotising them before the show to do various things on command on-air.

What first changed my mind about hypnosis was when Leon made Eleni (who is very petite) as stiff as a board and then balanced her horizontally between two chairs. Despite standing on her with his entire body weight, she remained still and completely rigid until he brought her out of the hypnosis.

My second experience was with Peter Powers, who once again spent a considerable amount of time hypnotising three members of my crew beforehand. On camera he made them all do some very funny things, but what really won me over on this occasion was Peter convincing Jason to eat an onion thinking he was biting into a juicy apple. He was merrily munching away enjoying it, Tony Abbott style, and only when Peter snapped him out of it after he'd eaten a good quarter of the onion did he spit the rest out and feel his mouth burning and needing something to cool it down.

My first time being hypnotised came during my last *Susie* show in 2008 when I invited Peter Powers to see if he could help me overcome what was often a debilitating fear of heights. We went to the top of the Sydney Tower, which is twice the height of the Sydney Harbour Bridge.

I was already hyperventilating just looking up from the street and certainly couldn't even get close to the glass on the observation deck, so I was terrified how I was going to get out onto the outdoor glass platform, 450 metres above Pitt Street.

Peter was at a wedding in Queensland the night before and his plane was delayed so he didn't have as much time to hypnotise me as he'd spent on my crew on previous shows, but much to my surprise I still responded very well.

I obeyed all his commands and was conscious of everything he said and asked me to do, and was stunned when he said I was ready because I didn't feel like I was hypnotised.

However, I did feel different. It was like I was wearing an invisible protective shield that emanated calmness. I wasn't nervous when put into the special suit you must wear and harnessed onto a special rail and to my utter astonishment I wasn't panicking while waking out onto the glass platform or looking down.

Ordinarily I would have been clinging to the side rails trying to control my breathing and doing everything not to look down to avoid freaking out and having a full-on anxiety attack. Instead, I was looking around and down very calmly and expressing how amazed I was that I could be out there doing this. Scotty McRae was a regular on my show and had joined me on camera throughout the show for support. We all posed for photos on the glass platform but when he suggested we do a Toyota style jump each time there was no way I could convince myself to go that next step. I mentioned that to Peter Powers and he said that in such a small amount of time he'd only been able to take me under very lightly.

At the time he also hypnotised me to do a two-finger movement squeezing my thumb and middle finger together if I'm ever overwhelmed by my height phobia again I've found that reduces the severity immediately. Overall, Peter's hypnosis has reduced my once debilitating fear of heights down to a very cautious respect for heights that's made it so much easier to manage.

The third hypnotist to impress me was Mark Stephens. Mark is a master practitioner of hypnosis, an accredited NLP trainer, has a black belt in martial arts and is the author of *Think Slim and Think Quit* (Allen & Unwin). He generously gave up his sleep many times to speak live to-air on my talkback radio show and share his tips on overcoming our phobias and addictions through meditation and hypnotherapy.

Mark's biggest success story is Jordon from Dulwich Hill in Sydney, who needed a weighbridge to tell him he weighed over 300 kilograms and who has now shed over 200 kilograms. Mark Stephens was the first to tell me about virtual gastric band hypnosis before I was able to try it for myself.

That all came about in September 2015 when I was asked by *New Idea* to appear on the cover of their magazine in a bikini as Kerri-Anne Kennerley had recently done on the cover of *Woman's Day*. I told them I wished my body looked as good as Kerri-Anne's and if it ever did I'd even pose nude for *Playboy!*

What I also confessed was that I'd stacked three or four dress sizes back on again and wouldn't be photographed in a one-piece costume, let alone a bikini. They offered to send me to a hypnotherapist and see if that made a difference to me shedding those excess kilos again and I jumped at the opportunity.

They arranged for me to see hypnotherapist Tim Thornton in Macquarie Street in Sydney and he started our six hypnotherapy sessions taking me through the virtual gastric band procedure as though you were actually going into the operating theatre.

The treatment was very successful, I had my first session late on Melbourne Cup day and then weekly and fortnightly sessions after that and I didn't overindulge for the first time during Christmas and New Year.

What kept me on the straight and narrow was Tim's eating plan, which was almost the same as Dr Gary Fettke's LCHF – Low Carbs Healthy Fats – food fuel.

As soon as I started eating refined sugar again and the receptors in my brain were flooded with feel good endorphins it became harder and harder to counteract these cravings with the follow-up audio tapes from Tim and Mark.

As I discussed in Chapter 3 'We are what we eat', refined sugar is not only a corrosive that can rust out our insides and gives us health issues such as type 2 diabetes, it also has the ability to change the chemicals in our brain that make us crave it like an addictive drug.

## Reverse negative thinking

From past experience, I've found it's never taken me long after negative thinking takes up rent-free space in my head for my brain-box to start sending dodgy signals that head straight to my stomach, demanding I fill it with lots of comfort food, which of course is always filled with fat and sugar.

I've sometimes even gone into a trance-like state while eating and before I knew it I'd have unconsciously consumed an entire packet/s of Tim Tams or Kettle chips.

This was the sort of reactionary behaviour that had to change if I wanted to maintain my dream car size and shape. My mind's computer had to be rebooted and reprogrammed to rid myself of the corrupted files in my brain that were making me fall back into my bad old habits. I had to download a few new apps to start responding differently to stressful situations whenever I'd hit a roadblock or went off-road on my life's journey.

One of the 'human auto-electricians', who specialises in the mind is master neuro linguistic programming trainer and psychotherapist Laureli Blyth.

Laureli is based in Sydney and her work takes her to the Asia Pacific, Europe, the UK and the US. She's authored five books and been voted by her peers as one of the top 30 global gurus of NLP.

There was never any shortage of callers into my overnight talkback radio show whenever Laureli would stop by to pass on some wonderful NLP techniques to help my listeners transcend their limiting thoughts and negative emotions and behaviours. I've once again drawn on Laureli Blyth's NLP expertise and generosity to share her sage advice in this book.

**Susie:** What is NLP? How can it benefit us?

**Laureli:** Neuro Linguistic Programming (NLP) is understanding how the language of your mind creates the programs of your life. NLP contains skills and knowledge that allows you to identify how the programs were created, how to enhance the programs that work well, how to change what doesn't work well to be able to create the programming you desire to have.

    The benefits of NLP are very useful as a communication and personal development tool. It allows you to understand more about yourself, grow, change and align your programming. NLP has a set of tools and techniques that are useful for many unwanted habits such as eating disorders, procrastination, laziness, and any negative behaviours and habits that you don't want.

    There are also methods to collapse the anchors of whatever is triggering the behaviour or habit, and tools to set and achieve goals. NLP teaches how to maintain your mind and how to create new programs and patterns that are in alignment with the life you want to have.

**Susie:** What steps can we take to overcome negative thinking?

**Laureli:** The mere idea that you will change negative thinking does not create change by itself. To create a new thought pattern you need to build a pathway to show and tell the brain/mind how to do it. In other words, create a new mental map in the brain and change the neuroplasticity with conscious intention.

    Sigmund Freud said 'In the beginning words and magic were one and the same.' The words and language we use are a very real indicator of the degree to which we project ourselves. These words become self-fulfilling prophecies. Things said in jest or in habit go into our unconscious mind where they become direct commands for our mind to actualise them.

    Think of how many times you say seemingly harmless comments to yourself such as 'I'm not good at doing that,' or 'My memory is not good,' or 'I'm so tired of this.' You are literally programming how you think and feel about yourself and your life. What would happen if instead you said, 'I will start thinking about it now'? Or 'I do know, I'm working on it now.'

Learn how to speak and direct your life with the words that will enhance your life. When you do this you relate to yourself and communicate with others with inspirational language. It has been recognised that positive reinforcement and proactive words can change the structure of our brain. Remember: words and language work whether they are positive or negative.

There is a great quote by author and motivational humourist Al Walker that says 'The most important words you will ever utter are those you say to yourself, about yourself, when you are by yourself.' This is such a powerful statement – our internal dialogue is a guide for our lives, and you cannot turn it off. What you can do however, is manage your thoughts, your mind and your internal dialogue.

**Susie:** Do our thoughts over time become our habits?

**Laureli:** The mind is very ritualistic in many ways, and works best with habits and routines; in fact, habits are very easy to create – but not always as easy to change! Often, we hear people say they continue with the old unwanted habit or behaviour because they don't know what they would rather do, they don't have the willpower or resolve to change or they have tried but it didn't work. We know that recurring thoughts over time do become our behaviours and habits. Because you are writing your internal code constantly based on how you think, feel, respond to the world, it can only produce results that will affect how your life is experienced.

There is a quote that comes from the Taoist philosopher Lao Tzu that Mahatma Gandhi often used. It shows that people have been aware long before science could validate neural pathways in humans: 'Your beliefs become your thoughts, your thoughts become your words, your words become your actions, your actions become your habits, your habits become your values and your values become your destiny.' Knowing this makes me curious why so many people don't seriously manage their thoughts first in order to change their habits.

**Susie:** How can we clear the clutter that blocks the communication connection between the conscious mind and unconscious mind?

**Laureli:** First of all let me clarify what we mean when we talk about the conscious and unconscious mind. The conscious mind is thought to make up only 10 per cent of our mind – it is responsible for thinking, analysing, judging and reasoning. While you may think it is your conscious mind that is in charge of you because you may be so aware of its incessant chatter, this isn't the case. Your unconscious mind makes up the other 90 per cent of your mind, also known as the subconscious or non-conscious mind, it is really this part of you that runs your body. It also stores your memories, creates your emotions, creates and transmits chemicals and is responsible for every part of your life. It is your unconscious mind that is responsible for organising and using your programs and patterns of emotion, thoughts, beliefs and behaviour. If you've ever tried to think your way into health or happiness, you'll know that your conscious mind isn't responsible for such things. It is your unconscious mind that needs to be rewired. In fact you never really solve a problem by thinking about it. The answers always come when you let it go and let your unconscious mind send through solutions.

The clutter or negative thoughts block the clear-thinking thoughts as you have no space to contemplate them. It is said you can't hold a thought of hope and worry at the same time. The difference between someone who gets overloaded with their own thoughts and someone who does not is simply what they pay attention to. When you know better you can do better and learning to manage your internal thoughts is a life-changing skill that everyone should know and learn to use.

**Susie:** Tell us about mindful thinking and living with intention?

**Laureli:** I've used mindfulness for over 30 years. It is a state of being in the present moment, including an awareness of thought but without any attachment; you are just noticing. Mindful thinking creates a space between thoughts and actions. It helps to break old habits or the knee-jerk reactions to things that happen in your life. Some people think it's meditating, but it's not, although it may help you keep your cool throughout the day! What it will help is to expand your own awareness about yourself and others around you.

Being more mindful has been correlated to a greater sense of wellbeing, happiness and health. When you are more present and mindful in the moment worry, anxiety, depression and illness can diminish; leaving you in the moment with more awareness of right here and right now.

Being mindful and living with intention is a great skill to build. What I do is set at least four mindful times a day for up to 78 seconds a time. For instance, when I am brushing my teeth, before I eat lunch, before I leave work for home, and before I go to bed. I stop for those moments and become aware and tune into the moment and the world around. I say, 'Here I am now, at this place, doing this thing, breathing seeing, being me.' I look forward to those times as my gems of the day.

When you can create a habit of mindfulness unresourceful emotions and behaviours have a harder time of penetrating your now. You will be more aware of your interactions in the world and more choices will become available to you.

**Susie:** What are ways to get in and stay in a positive mindset?

**Laureli:** There is a saying 'energy goes where your attention flows', that is, where we put our focus is what we bring into our lives, or the law of attraction. Ultimately, the law of attraction says that we are able to influence our lives by directing our thoughts to what we want instead of what we don't want. NLP takes this concept a few steps further with more understanding of how the unconscious mind works and also how we can sabotage those efforts by outdated programming. When we know this and use our mind to focus on what we want versus what we don't want, amazing things happen.

For some people they think if they don't mull over what could go wrong first then they may not be prepared. There is nothing wrong with having a Plan B, however, it's what you focus on and the story you run in your mind that programs how your life unfolds. For example, a person may really want to lose weight, get in shape and feel better, but if they have a pattern of not wanting to be noticed, or they keep thinking and saying to themselves that losing weight is hard, they will find it challenging to lose weight. Because that is what they are directing their mind to create.

What we think truly does affect what we believe and what we do; what we believe affects what we do and what we think; and what we do affects what we think about what we believe. It takes awareness to notice your thoughts and what you are paying attention to and then switch your thoughts and concentration onto what you do want. It does require your attention but it won't take long if you just do it.

**Susie:** How much of a part does nutrition play in our body's mind-body-spirit being in tune and functioning together?

**Laureli:** Whatever your mindset, emotional ties and beliefs are about food, they are the basis of your relationship with food. At the end of the day, food is just sustenance and fuel for the body, but we humans often put more meaning on it than just fuel. We get emotional about food. Over the years research has shown that your brain needs a balanced diet with nutrients, vitamins and supplements. But it also needs exercise and plenty of oxygen, hydration and relaxation. Without these essentials, brain cells are not efficient and memory and motor functions are impaired. To boost your memory and protect your brain cells you need to consume a diet rich in antioxidants. That means lots of vegetables, fruits, nuts, fish, seeds and supplements of vitamins A, C and E.

**Susie:** Please explain one of your favourite quotes, 'Knowledge is only a rumour until it is in the muscle.'

**Laureli:** The beautiful saying comes from the Asaro tribe of Indonesia and Papua New Guinea. To me this means that unless you do it, try it on, then it is not real for you. Too often people think they 'know' because they've read or heard or saw something, but to truly know you need to do experience it. This brings me to another favourite quote by the late Jimi Hendrix: 'Knowledge speaks and wisdom listens.' So be a wise listener to people who do know, but then try it on.

'Problems are not stop signs, they are guidelines'
- ROBERT SCHULLER

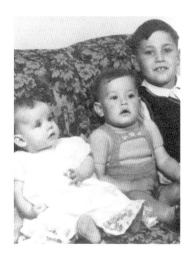

Left: Susie as a baby with her two brothers Eddie & Leon in 1954.

Centre: Susie and her brother Eddie at Pre-school in 1957. 'Despite Eddie being fifteen months older than me we were always thought of as twins.'

Bottom: Susie's brother Leon celebrates his 21st birthday. From left to right: Mum, Dad, Leon, Susie (age 14 and size 14) & Eddie.

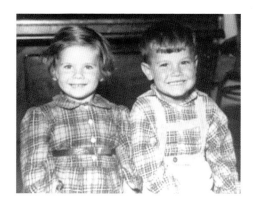

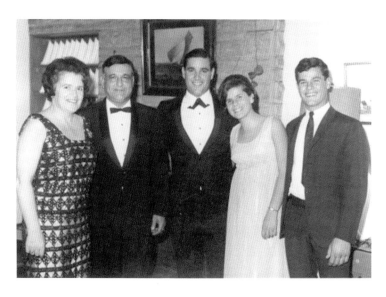

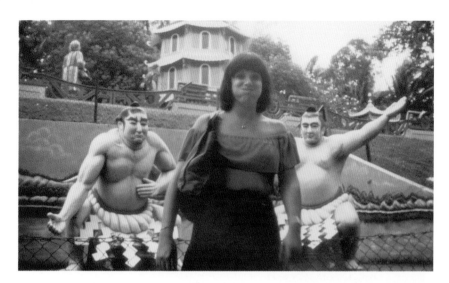

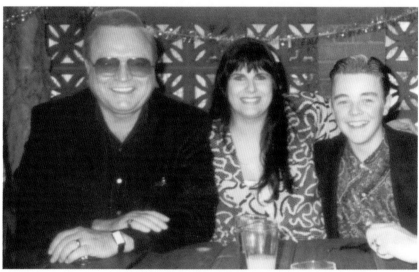

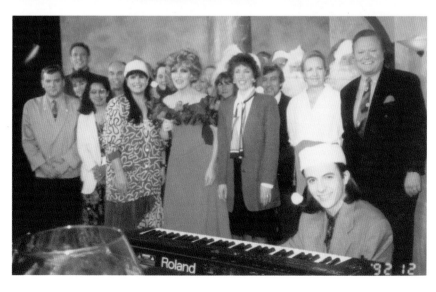

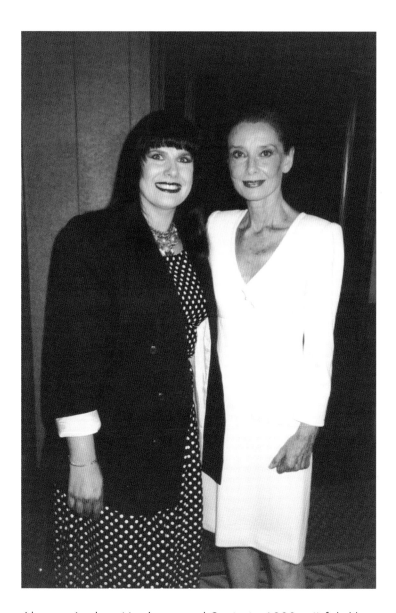

Above: Audrey Hepburn and Susie in 1989 – 'I felt like such a frump alongside Audrey, she was so elegant and graceful and lean'.

Opposite page from top: Susie in Singapore in the late 70s – 'We could be mistaken for triplets.' Centre: Susie with Bert Newton and Matthew Newton in 1992. 'Bert wasn't the only Moonface here.' Bottom: *Good Morning Australia* Christmas Show 1992 – 'Not hard to spot me, that outfit was size 22 and I'm standing next to Jeanne Little who looks a quarter of my size.'

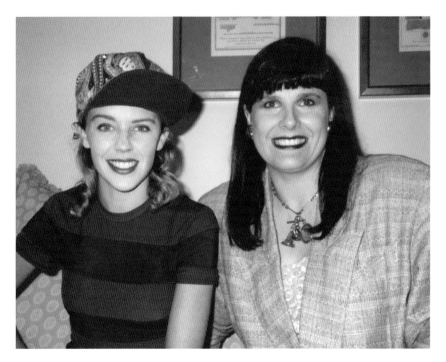

Kylie Minogue and Susie in 1989 – 'I think we've both improved with age.'

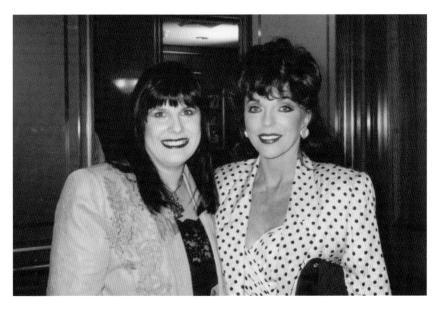

Joan Collins and Susie in 1989 – 'Joan was almost twice my age and half my size.'

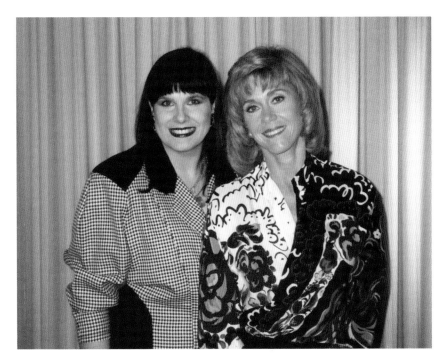

Above: Jane Fonda and Susie in 1989 – 'Half my body is hidden behind Jane, who looked fantastic.'

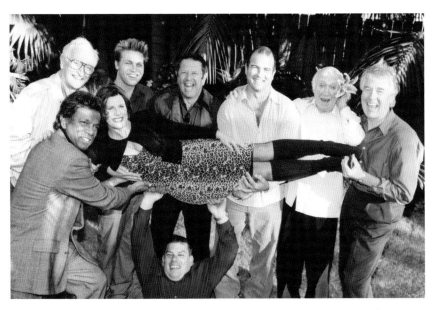

Below: Launch of 'Susie & the Blokes' on 2GB, at Bernard King's home, from left to right: Kamahl, Stuart Wagstaff, Nathan Harvey, George Smilovici, James Blundell, Bernard King, Col Joye and underneath me doing most of the work is John Coutis.

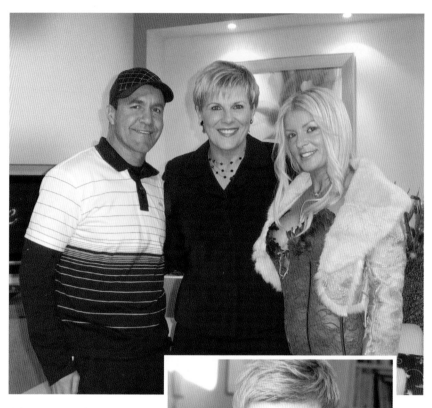

2007 – 'Nothing made me fitter or changed my shape more than boxing training with Jeff Fenech. Jeff and his wife Suzee are both fantastic trainers.

PHOTO COURTESY OF THE WIN-TV NETWORK

PHOTO: CYBELE MALINOWSKI

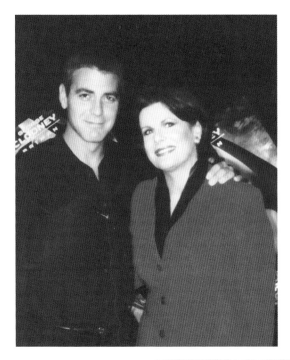

George Clooney and Susie in 1997 – 'George invited me to sit on his lap, but I told him I thought I'd probably break it if I did.'

Susie snorkelling off Hayman Island in the late 90s – 'No matter how much weight I've shed I still have those terrible internal saddle bags just like my Mum.'

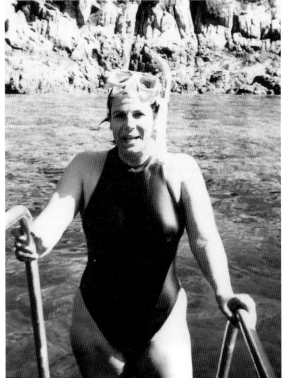

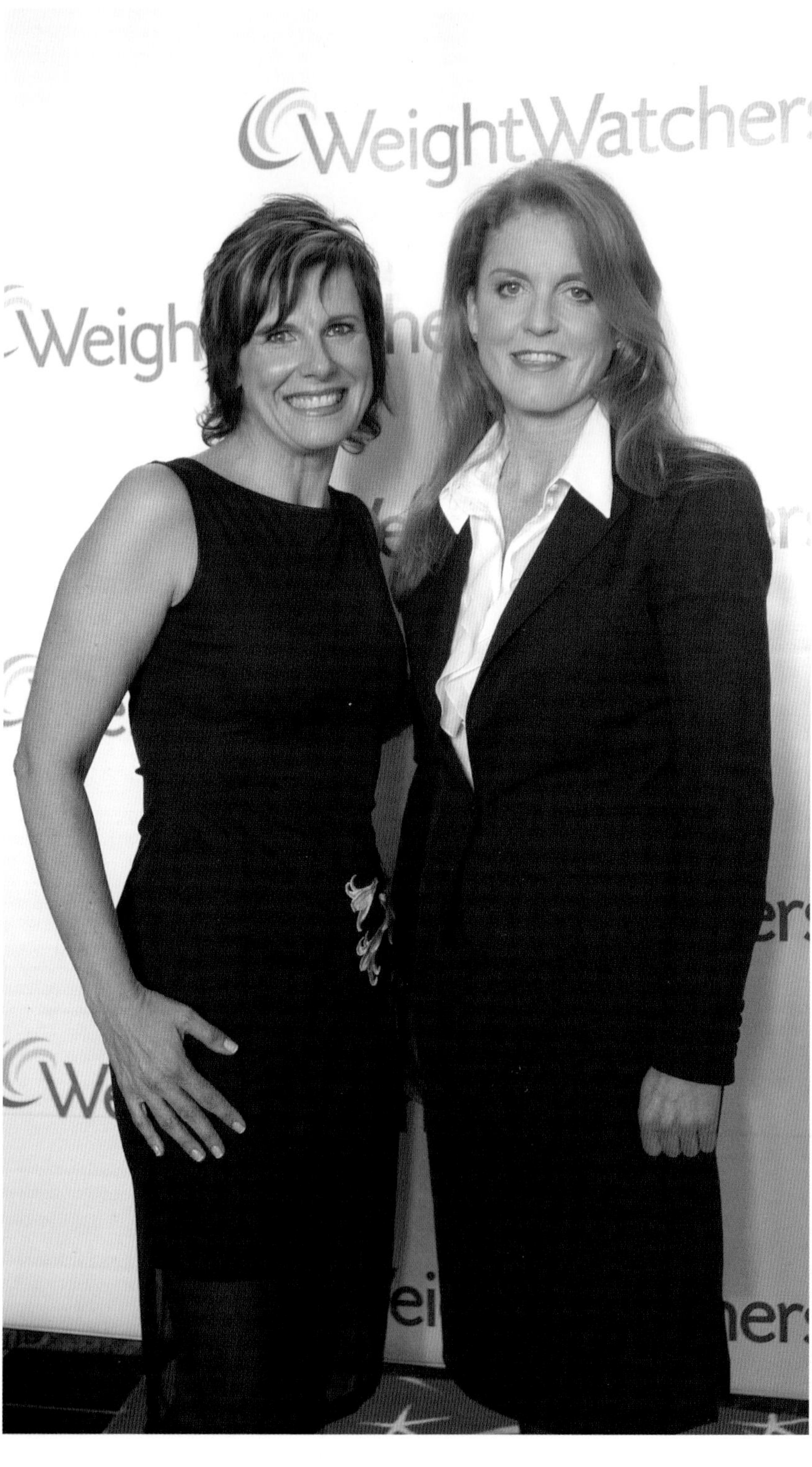
WeightWatchers

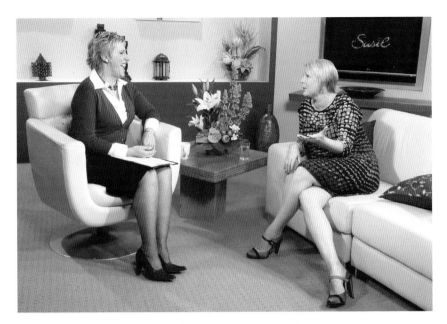

In 2008 with the divine Julia Morris on set during my national variety and lifestyle TV show *SUSIE*. Read why we admire each other's willpower on page 128.

PHOTO COURTESY OF THE WIN-TV NETWORK

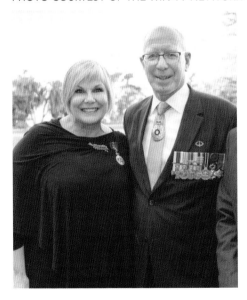

In 2015 humbly receiving my AM – Medal of the Order of Australia – from New South Wales Governor David Hurley. I was off the rails again with my emotions and comfort eating and recovering from another foot operation.

PHOTO COURTESY OF ROB TUCKWELL PHOTOGRAPHY

Opposite page: Sarah Ferguson, the Duchess of York, and Susie in March 2003 at the Weight Watchers Super Rally at Fox Studios – 'Sarah is an inspiration!'

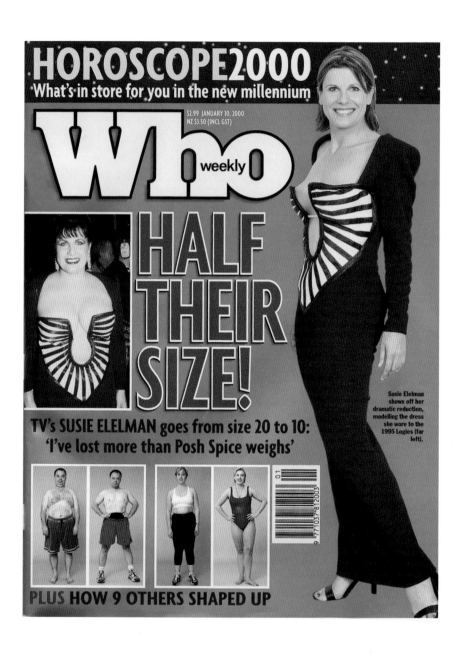

Who magazine, 'Half My Size' cover, January 10, 2000.

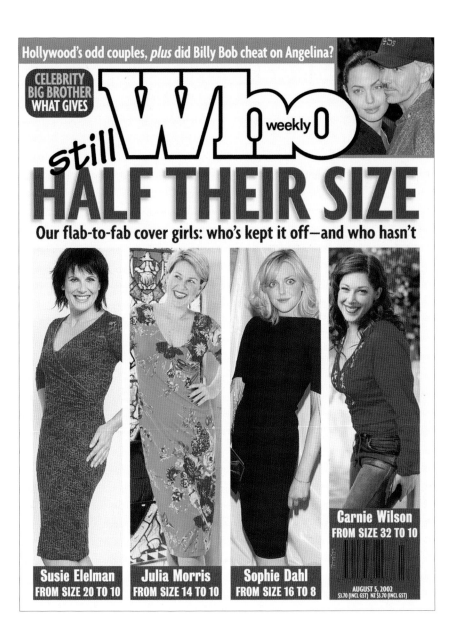

Hollywood's odd couples, *plus* did Billy Bob cheat on Angelina?

CELEBRITY
BIG BROTHER
WHAT GIVES

# Who weekly

## *still* HALF THEIR SIZE

Our flab-to-fab cover girls: who's kept it off—and who hasn't

**Susie Elelman**
FROM SIZE 20 TO 10

**Julia Morris**
FROM SIZE 14 TO 10

**Sophie Dahl**
FROM SIZE 16 TO 8

**Carnie Wilson**
FROM SIZE 32 TO 10

AUGUST 5, 2002
$3.70 (INCL GST)  NZ $3.70 (INCL GST)

*Who* magazine, 'Still Half My Size' cover, August 5, 2002.

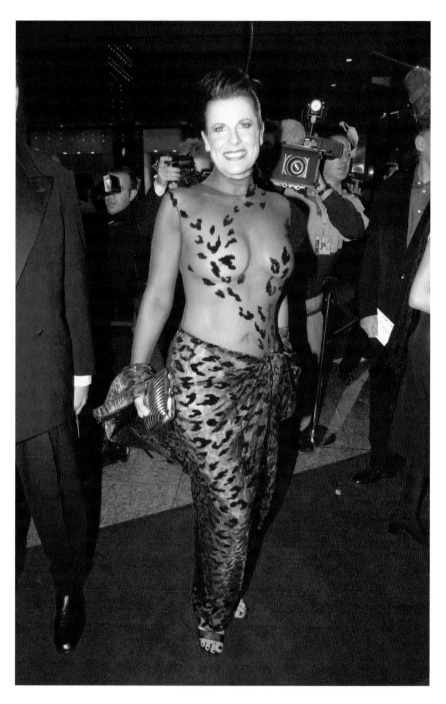

Susie at the Logie Awards 2001 – 'This is still my favourite Logies outfit. An amazing Christopher Essex creation that defies gravity. I didn't exhale all night.' PHOTO COURTESY OF BELINDA ROLLAND

Right: Susie at the Logie Awards 2003 – 'Another work of art by Christopher Essex.'

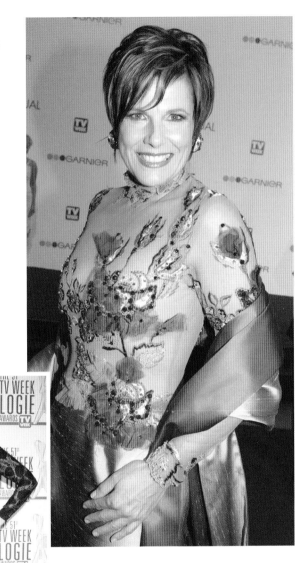

At the 2009 Logies I was excited to fit back into my vintage Covers lace body suit from the 1980s, which I teamed up with a stunning red skirt I found in an Op Shop.

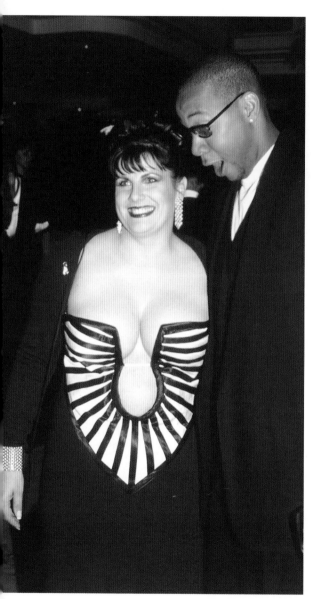

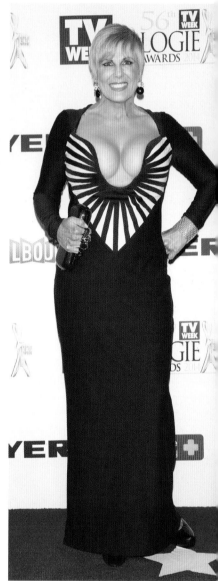

Left: Susie with US Comedian Mark Curry. I still love this 1995 Logie gown but I hated the body in it. I was twice my size and made Who Weekly's Worst Dressed list for the first time. PHOTO COURTESY *TV WEEK*
Right: To celebrate 40 years in TV and turning 60 I asked dressmaker/designer Peter Bartlett to replicate that 1995 dress. It received very mixed reactions. Depending on my pose, from certain angles the stripes caused an optical illusion in photographs.
PHOTO COURTESY *TV WEEK*

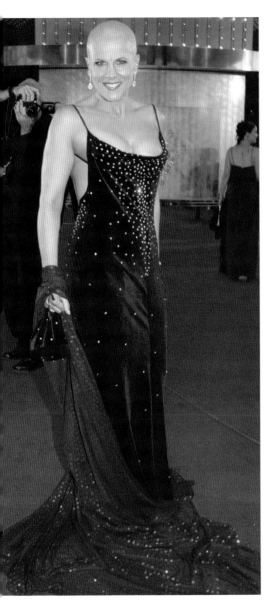
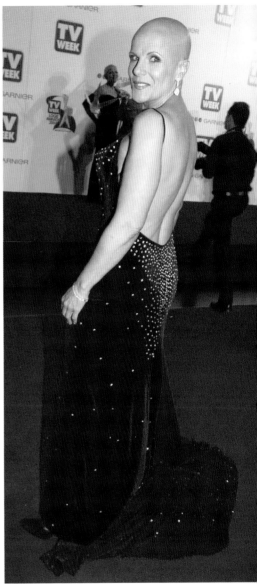

Susie at the Logie Awards in 2004 – 'This stunning Christopher Essex gown was somewhat overshadowed by me shaving my head, which I did to celebrate 30 years in TV and turning 50 years of age. A well known TV presenter came up to me that night and said "I'm 30 and I hope I look that good at 50!" I thanked her and replied, "I wished I looked this good at 30!"'

PHOTO LEFT COURTESY *TV WEEK*
PHOTO RIGHT COURTESY OF BELINDA ROLLAND

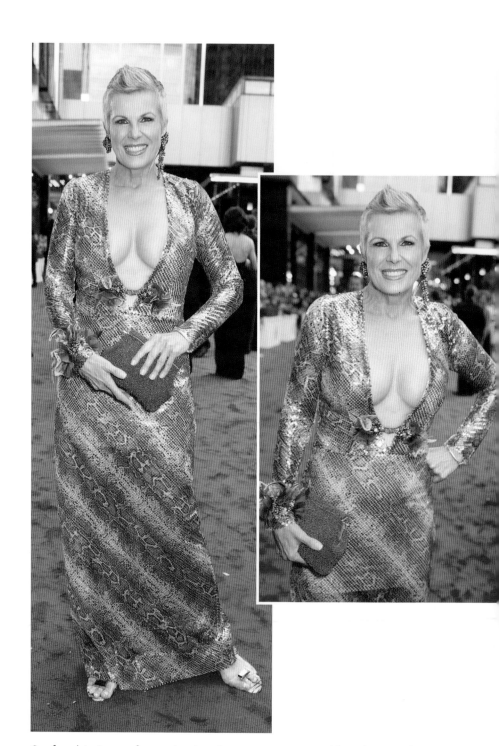

So far this is my favourite Logies gown, created by dressmaker/
designer Peter Bartlett in 2013. PHOTO COURTESY *TV WEEK*

# Willpower tips from celebrity lips

**Susie:** What do like most about your body?

**Trevor Hendy:** I like the balance of my body. It's not a question that a guy gets asked very often.

**Shelley Taylor-Smith:** I like my breasts because they survived my cancer scare. My body has amazed me. It's never let me down. It has always come through and you better bloody well listen to it and respect your body as you're only here for a short time so it better be a bloody good time. So enjoy it!

**Sandra Sully:** Not much really, but if I had to choose, my arms and my stomach, although don't look too closely!!

**Wayne Pearce:** Abs, I suppose.

**Tara Moss:** It functions. I know people whose don't, so I am grateful I've got all my bits and pieces and I do hope they stick around for a while.

**Fran Macpherson:** I'm tall. I love height. It's more about how you feel about yourself personally, than what your weight is. You have to like yourself, be happy with how you live your life.

**Jessica Rowe:** I like that my body's strong.

**Susie:** Do you have strong willpower?

**Tara Moss:** I'm not methodical but I'm extremely motivated and I think that's enough. As long as you are motivated and you're intelligent about what your motivations are, you will make out okay in life.

**Wayne Pearce:** I think there's a genetic component to willpower, but I think a lot of it is also to do with the success that you have when you're younger that fuels the desire for more success. Once you've had a little bit of success you realise how good you feel about yourself, probably with the weight loss as well, therefore you want more success. The downside, I suppose, of having strong willpower is that you run the risk of becoming too consumed in a particular goal or passion in life to the point where your life loses balance and a sense of focus.

**Susie:** Is it hard to say no to fatty foods?

**Wayne Pearce:** It's just what you are used to, what you become conditioned to and that's where the value is of affirming to yourself what you want in life, what are your priorities. I look at a food and think 'There are a lot of nutrients in that food. It's not too high or low glycaemic index, I'd like to have that,' or I do the opposite if I think it's not such a good food. But not everybody consciously thinks that way about food.

**Susie:** Can you give me some tips on how you can overcome the mental obstacles that prevent you from reaching your goals and values?

**Wayne Pearce:** I think visualisation and affirmation are the two keys. Visualisation is very powerful; you have to see yourself as you want to be when you look in the mirror. In your own mind you have to create an image of what you want to be like and you have to see that image on a regular basis, and if you do that you can reprogram your subconscious to draw you towards where you want to be. Visualisation works from a visual angle, affirmation works from a thinking angle – when I say to myself that I am capable of being fit, healthy and slim or I am capable of having a slim figure.

**Jeff Fenech:** If you get your priorities right, everything else will fall into place. Preparation. Mentally prepare for the task ahead. Physically be ready for the challenge.

**Tara Moss:** It really is about doing it. I think the biggest tragedy in life is not giving it a go. I've got at least a thousand failures under my belt. Everyone I know who is successful has some colossal failures under their belt. Prepare, be persistent and one day the opportunity will come. Whether that's in twenty years or tomorrow, you don't know. You've got to be ready.

# CHAPTER 6

# FAIL TO PLAN: PLAN TO FAIL

'An objective, without a plan is a dream.'
- DOUGLAS MCGREGOR

By now I'm hoping you are feeling excited, comfortable and in control, sitting in the driver's seat of your dream car, or soon to be dream car. Maybe you're feeling like you'd be happier in the passenger seat; that's okay too. It's a great start but eventually you'll have to mentally get behind the wheel to truly take control of your own journey and destination. And if you're going to be a passenger for now, remember how important it is not to turn into a backseat driver. Are you ready? Please get comfortable, adjust your seat and backrest, check your rear and side vision mirrors and fasten your seatbelt because you could be in for a bumpy ride.

Hopefully Chapter 3 'We are what we eat' has helped you work out your optimum food fuel mix and Chapter 4 'Get your motor running' has given you interesting ways to get moving and shown you how you can get into top gear without blowing a head gasket and there's more fuel burning tips in Chapter 11 'Add SEX and double your result!'

The next step is to arm you with the mental tools to keep you on track and make you feel charged, ready and raring to go.

I use the electrical system on a car as the best motoring analogy to describe my emotional system. And I'll be the first to acknowledge that my mind's engine isn't always firing on all cylinders. Many things can trigger it to short-circuit or overheat. Sometimes it's not something your local GP can fix; it might require a referral to the human equivalent of an auto electrician. This chapter highlights how to use some of the items in your easy-to-use kit, which you'll find neatly tucked up in the human glove box – your brain – for easy access to help keep your willpower revs up.

## The journey ahead

'If you don't know where you are going, every road will get you nowhere.'
- HENRY KISSINGER

Where do we begin? I think it's vital to have aims and ambitions and to understand the reason why you want to achieve them. When you have a purpose and put your goals sturdily in place, you can draw on the end game as strength when your willpower or motivation starts to wane. Next is to put a plan in place to make it all come to fruition.

Goal setting is a major tool in achieving anything you want in life. Whether it's to improve your body image, buy a property, travel overseas or learn to play a musical instrument. Yearning for a better relationship with your partner and family is one thing, but it's the goals you set in place and follow through with that turn those dreams into reality. Goals give clarity, definition and direction to our aims.

Please don't confuse wishing with goal setting. I wish I was a multi-millionaire but if I look at this realistically, I wouldn't be able to earn that sort of money doing my current occupations, I don't buy lottery tickets so I'll never become an instant winner and I don't have any rich relatives whose fortune I will inherit. I can wish all I like but the only way I'm ever going to accomplish my financial

STILL HALF MY SIZE

aspirations is to set achievable goals and then utilise my talent and skills to make them happen.

Do you set goals and then work towards them? Or do you find goal setting puts you in a position of conflict – either with yourself, or maybe your partner or an employer? Or do you just drift through life with a go-with-the-flow attitude, not wanting to feel locked into a plan? A person with this sort of attitude can still set goals.

If you're not used to goal setting please don't be scared. May I suggest you start with small daily goals so you can get used to working towards bigger goals and to seeing the results. For instance, your goal tomorrow might be to find time to exercise, or to get up ten minutes earlier and have breakfast, or to clean out your wardrobe, or to practise a musical instrument you've been learning. Your goal might be to meet someone new. Simply finding time for yourself can be one of the hardest goals to achieve yet one of the most important. Whatever purpose you want to fulfil, put goals in place to achieve it.

Some goals are short-term and others long-term but goals must have a timeframe … otherwise they are still just dreams. Some goals, once achieved, can be ticked off the list. Others, like maintaining your new size and shape, will require a lifetime of regularly drawing on the various tools you now have at your disposal in your glove box to continue to achieve this success.

Make sure you set goals that you can realistically achieve. I'm not saying don't aim high. Quite the contrary, one of my favourite sayings is by Norman Vincent Peale, the US Minister, radio broadcaster and author of many self-help books including *The Power of Positive Thinking*. He said, 'Shoot for the moon, even if you miss, you'll land among the stars.' There is, however, a big difference between high hopes and pie-in-the-sky ideas that are too far out of reach, have no foundation for success and are, therefore, often doomed to fail before you start.

Just like the get-rich-quick schemes that always sound too good to be true, mainly because they are too good to be true, there's no quick fix in weight management and shedding stored body fat and keeping if off; it requires permanent lifestyle changes.

The long-term goal I set for myself when I was a size 20 was to get back down to a size 14. The main reason for this was so that I could walk back into most shops and be able pick something off the rack and have it fit me. The benefits of achieving any goal are endless and far-reaching. In my case, getting down to a size 14 not only made me look and feel better about myself, it opened up so many more opportunities. I was once again within the size range of many wonderful dress designers and suddenly found I had an enormous variety of stunning labels that I could fit into. For the first time in many years I could choose how I wanted to dress, rather than dressing to cover my size. Not to mention the fact that I could fit into so many more of the great clothes I already owned but hadn't worn for years.

## Check your street directory occasionally

'Fortune is a prize to be won. Adventure is the road to it.
Chance is what may lurk in the shadows of the roadside.'
– O HENRY

Once you've reached your goal, you can always raise the bar a bit higher. Reviewing your results is vital. When I reached a size 14, I was so happy that I forgot about my size and embarked on another goal. That was to maintain what I had achieved through a lifestyle change of a healthy fuel mix and continued exercise. Before I knew it I was down to a size 12 and then through other emotional and health issues even further to a size 8–10. I think I've only been that size once before in my adult life and I didn't stay there for very long back then and I was about to do the same again.

I can proudly say I've outdone my own expectations and reset my goals once again; One has been to firm and tone my chassis; shedding such an enormous amount of weight, and more than once, has unfortunately left my duco with some severe hail damage in spots and my upholstery sagging in other spots that were once filled with my stored body fat. Rather than going off to the panel beater to have expensive cosmetic surgery, I've chosen the more affordable DIY approach of old-fashioned sit-ups and light weights.

## Stay focused

It's important that I keep up my long-term maintenance plan to ensure that I don't slip back into my old ways. The last thing I ever want is to be steering around an eighteen-wheeler again.

One thing's for sure, change can push me out of my comfort zone and often causes me uncomfortable emotions of fear and panic and the feeling of being out of control. Consciously taking deep breaths and then slowly releasing them helps to calm me as I try to examine what's frightening me and figure out how to overcome the problem. I'm a big believer in the power of positive thinking and that you'll stand to achieve far more by continually reinforcing your aspirations and optimistic mindset than you will by being plagued with negative thoughts.

Understandably, when it comes to maintaining our body vehicles, we won't always be able to motor comfortably along life's road. I'm trying, however, to ensure that I have systems in place that prevent me from finding myself hanging on, white knuckled, to the front handlebar of another wild roller-coaster ride.

Extending ourselves is exciting but it can also make us want to retreat back and stay comfortably where we are instead of moving forward, embracing the change and reaping the benefits. As adults we must take control of our own destiny.

## Keep your goals clearly in sight

Think of your goals as dreams with a deadline. Write them down, hang them up, and watch them happen. John McGrath, author of *The Most Valuable Lessons I Have Learned* has a novel way of keeping his long- and short-term goals and objectives right before his eyes: he laminates them and sticks them up in the shower and on the bathroom mirror.

I've noticed another friend has the goals that excite him crawling across his computer as his screen saver. I keep them on my fridge door with magnets. Maybe you have some innovative methods of your own. Put them on a wall or a door in the toilet – anywhere you'll see them regularly.

## Susie's goal-setting tips

- Be clear about your goals

- Start small and with easy ones

- Raise the bar higher as you have successes

- Prioritise your goals

- Implement a simple action plan and a deadline for each one

- Follow it daily

- Review your results

- Change direction if necessary

- Stay focused

- Be positive and believe in yourself

# Procrastination

Which lane of life are you in at the moment? Are you parked in a rest bay? Or maybe you're the slow poke towing that big caravan up a steep, windy mountain road? I find the singer Joan Baez's quote a poignant reminder about how I should be living life: 'You don't get to choose how you're going to die or when. You can only decide how you're going to live. Now!' The US humourist Don Marquis describes procrastination as the art of keeping up with yesterday.

In Dr Stephen R Covey's best-selling book *The 7 Habits of Highly Effective People* the first of his habit is to be proactive. Do you usually say 'Oh I'll start my diet on Monday'? Or, 'I won't start thinking about a diet until after so and so's birthday'? What are you waiting for? For years a friend of mine used to say, in relation to bills, 'I'll pay it tomorrow!' Now he pays every bill within five minutes of opening it because he used to forget them and get himself into a lot of trouble. He's decided that 'Do it now!' is so much simpler emotionally.

Dr Covey's second habit is to always have the end in mind. My goal is to look and feel in good enough shape to be comfortable with the top down on my sleek '54 convertible Mercedes this summer … what's yours?

## Look out for the potholes

Unlike potholes in the road that cause trouble for our suspension when we hit them, food potholes are generally cushioned and disguised by their yummy taste. Food potholes don't jar our bodies when we encounter them; quite the contrary, the more we eat the more padding we develop. Before you know it the whole street is so littered with hazardous obstacles that you've gone completely off-road again. It's often easier to clear the trouble spots and get back on the straight and narrow by starting again and giving your road a total re-tarring.

It is so easy to come up with reasons and excuses to justify why we can't achieve our goals. If your best friend were to ask you why you were eating something and your reaction would be to stop eating it, or not to eat it at all, then be conscious of the times when you ask yourself the same question. Don't hide the question and don't rationalise or justify continuing to eat whatever it is. Be honest with yourself!

## Too busy

How often have we all been swallowed up into that bottomless 'too busy' pit? When you add all the blood, sweat and tears that we torrentially pour into the things that are making us too busy then the pit turns into a quagmire. We all have the same 24 hours in the day; it just depends what we choose to do with each of those 24 hours.

A great time management tip is the Three-D Principle. I learnt this from one of my greatest mentors, Doug Malouf, who was inarguably one of Australia's most brilliant public speakers, authors, and business educators. Dougie always taught me that you waste too much time if you are indecisive. Three-D Principle is to Do, Dump or Delegate. Whatever comes across your path, decide to either DO it, DUMP it or DELEGATE it.

Believe it or not, most of us find the hardest D to achieve is the last one – delegate. Remember that delegating isn't like dumping; you can still have control and follow-up but it also allows you to do the first of the Three-D Principles. It's easy for all of us to take on too much and then try to be all things to all people but we only end up disappointing ourselves.

## Lists

I find the best way to manage my time is to make lists. I'm a huge list maker and a recycler and am able to do both as I keep used envelopes and write my lists on the back of them. After following the Three-D Principle of Do, Dump or Delegate, put anything you need to achieve on that daily list, then prioritise and work through the most important or urgent things first. Even if something unexpected crops up, add it to the list before you decide if you're going to proceed with it. Then when you've done it, cross it off and move onto the next task.

It's so important to prioritise your goals and set them out on a daily plan of action. Do the most important things first and allocate the appropriate amount of time for each task. Don't forget to take note of the number of things you were able to complete, and take credit for those achievements. At the end of each day move the things not completed that day over to the list for the next day.

Making lists empties your head of the responsibility of forgetting something, and you can focus your full attention on the tasks at hand. Making a list for the next day just before you go to bed or just after dinner will also relax you because now tomorrow has a plan and you have clear goals to try and work towards completing.

Rather than trying to remember everything, I'm a great one for leaving prompts to jog my memory. For instance, I'll use the kitchen timer to remind me that I've put bottles in the freezer to cool quickly or I'll hang a pair of shoes in a shoe bag on the front door to remind me to get them repaired.

Another great Weight Watchers' tip is to go shopping with a list. A list means you've planned what you're going to eat. If you deviate from the list, please at least do yourself a favour and read the label before you decide to buy something. The bonus is that your shopping will work out cheaper because you won't have any spontaneous purchases. By the same token, if you're thinking that you don't have enough things to do with your time to make up a list; be aware that a simple thing like boredom can weaken your resolve – it's good to keep busy.

## Incidental eating

Even if my meals and snacks are under control I can easily get caught up in incidental eating, like picking at salted roasted nuts over a drink and indulging in the dips and finger food at parties and get-togethers. The ex-pig in me thought of a smorgasbord as 'hog heaven' and it used to be a licence for me to endlessly chow down. Now by choosing to eat (LCHF) Low Carbs, Healthy Fats and avoid refined sugar and most grains I've eliminated 90 per cent of those bad foods automatically. That means there's not going to be a lot that I've allowed myself to eat that will lure me at parties and social events.

To help lubricate my willpower I use another Weight Watchers' practice – I'll often eat at home first before I go to parties and other social gatherings, especially if I know the event is only going to be full of very tempting 'leaded' fuel. The time of the event will determine whether I eat a full meal before I go out or just a snack like some hummus with fresh veggies or avocado and tomato, or some fruit and a handful of raw unsalted nuts. It's much easier to say no and mean it on a full stomach.

## Think ahead

I have much greater success if I can plan ahead. If I've allowed time in my day to prepare and eat healthy food and to exercise then I'm clearly on track. If not, I can easily fall by the wayside by not having healthy choices, especially in the snack department, to fill my emptying fuel tank.

I try to ensure that my fridge and pantry are stocked up with healthier alternatives so I'm not tempted to take the quick fix and regret it afterwards. If I find I have lots of vegies to use up I'll make a big pot of healthy low-fat soup such as Fran Macpherson's delicious recipe in the back of this book. To save time I make the soup the night before when I'm preparing dinner and allow it to cook slowly for a long time and then cool overnight.

Freezing portions of this soup, or any leftover 'unleaded' dishes I've made for dinner, makes a quick and easy healthy alternative when time is my enemy – and I'm most likely to grab something unhealthy if I haven't planned ahead.

# Role models

I try to surround myself with positive, like-minded people. I draw on their experience and I'm not frightened to seek help, as you've no doubt already gathered from the line-up of talented contributors to my book.

Often, just verbalising our desires to others gives us a sense of commitment and can empower us to find the willpower to carry them out. My role models and mentors come from many fields in life but I know a lot of my early influences came from television.

Years ago I actually had the chance to interview one of my childhood idols when I wrote a series of columns on self-esteem, motivation and willpower for *Woman's Day* and the lifestyle editor Emma-Charlotte Brown sent me a fabulous book to review before interviewing the author. I couldn't believe my luck.

*Living Alone and Loving It* (Simon & Schuster) is the title of a brilliant book written by Barbara Feldon. If the author's name isn't familiar to you, Barbara Feldon played Agent 99 in the television series *Get Smart,* which ran for five seasons from 1965–69 and has been playing in re-runs somewhere around the world ever since. It is one of the funniest television comedy shows to come out of America and I still get a laugh if I see an episode today. It was exciting to interview Barbara from New York when she launched her book and we chatted for almost an hour.

I was an impressionable eleven-year-old when *Get Smart* debuted on Australian television and I didn't just watch it for the comedy. I also tuned in to see what Agent 99 was wearing, saying and doing. Her character was everything I epitomised: Agent 99 is tall, slim, beautiful, intelligent, witty, well-spoken, clever and at the same time humble. Despite the fact that in most episodes Agent 99 saves the day and her man, Agent 86 (generally from himself!), she never let him lose face.

We can get caught up with idolising these fictitious folk but if you have the opportunity to meet the actor who brings them to life you sometimes discover that they are totally different to their character. However, in this case, after chatting to the actor who brought Agent

99 so memorably to the small screen, it wasn't hard to see how much of that strength of character was in Barbara Feldon first and foremost.

Barbara revealed that she found herself living alone after a relationship impasse and she didn't realise it at the time but it has now turned out to be the most enriching and joyous period of her life. Reading Barbara's book gave me a real shift in paradigm. It equipped me with more confidence to also continue to live alone and love it.

One of her key messages is to nurture a glowing self-image that is not dependent on an admirer. Barbara's book addresses the practical as well as the emotional side of being solo; especially overcoming loneliness, which can often trigger low self-esteem and overeating.

I can't encourage you enough to read Barbara's book, especially if you are frightened in any way of getting behind the wheel of your dream car and exploring exciting adventures without any passengers. You might find yourself newly divorced or recently widowed and Barbara's book sets out lots of wonderful foundation stones that will give you the confidence to at least drive out of your garage by yourself.

'The most dangerous part of any car is how loose the nut is behind the wheel.'
— BILL ELELMAN

## The Duchess of York and Weight Watchers

One of the most inspiring people I have met in recent times has been Sarah Ferguson, the Duchess of York. I emceed the Weight Watchers' Super Rally at Fox Studios and Fergie, as she's affectionately known, was the special guest and I interviewed her on stage. Sadly, only the night before, her dad had passed away and she was only informed when her plane landed in Bangkok on her way to Sydney. Instead of returning home she chose instead to continue onto Australia to fulfil all her engagements.

Like her sister Jane, who lives in Sydney where we've met socially on many occasions, Sarah too is down to earth and very warm and friendly. No-one would ever have known from her smiling, friendly outward facade that she was experiencing such a horrible loss. But I guess it wasn't the first time that Fergie has had to put on a brave face in public.

Having weathered many a mocking media headline the world over, it was refreshing to see that Fergie has equipped her dream car with the perfect shield – a very good sense of humour. In hindsight (with pun unintended) Sarah, who looked fantastic, could now even make self-deprecating remarks about being the Duchess of Pork.

Unlike Sarah Ferguson, I'm not paid by Weight Watchers to endorse their program in this book; I recommend it because I know it's a realistic way of achieving your dream-car shape and maintaining its optimum performance. I must say, Weight Watchers today is a far cry from when they first started 40 plus years ago, when you had to eat liver once a week and weigh all your food. In fact Weight Watchers is far more lenient than I am with myself about what foods to eat. The simple system that Weight Watchers has now developed to keep track of your food fuel means you know exactly how many 'food treats' you can have and still maintain your dream car size and shape. This sensible eating and exercise plan can easily be sustained for years and not days like some fad diets.

For many years I emceed and interviewed all the national finalists in the Weight Watchers' Slimmer of the Year Awards, which they now call their Healthy Life Awards and every one of their stories moved me. They are all role models, who have the most inspiring stories about their own weight journeys and I always learnt heaps from them.

The 2004 South Australian finalist Sonia Thornton gave me her philosophy on losing versus shedding weight. Have you ever thought about what happens to the weight you lose? Every time I've lost weight it, it's found me again! Sonia quite rightly points out that to lose something implies that you want to find it again. She says that shedding your weight is more like a snake shedding its skin or a butterfly shedding its cocoon.

> 'The dictionary is the only place where success comes before work.'
> – ARTHUR BRISBANE

## Public humiliation

Nothing makes your self-esteem plummet quicker than a bruised ego and dented pride. The first time I felt publicly humiliated was in 1995 when I made the worst-dressed list in *Who* magazine. It followed my appearance in the now infamous black and white Logies dress, which I talk more about in Chapter 10 'Smoke & mirrors' and you can see photos in the photo gallery. Suddenly I became newspaper, magazine and current affairs' show fodder. They all wanted to interview me about it. I couldn't hide and I found all the negative publicity soul-destroying.

I made the same list again two years later but I then managed to right the scales of justice and get on the best-dressed list once, along with an honourable mention the following year. Over the following decades I've adorned the covers and taken up many single column centimetres in magazines and newspapers in relation to my size and shape and while a lot of it has been negative, I've now managed to turn it all around.

One of my proudest moments was in January 2000 when I made the cover of *Who* magazine's 'Half Their Size' issue, which turned out to be the biggest single selling issue that year. I wonder if me buying 4352 copies made any difference? Just kidding! I can remember walking into the Golden Wing Lounge at Sydney airport on my way up to the Golden Door Health Retreat with one of my close friends, Sherryl, and the lovely attendant at the counter said, 'Oh, these were just delivered, do you want to be the first to see it?'

With that he produced several copies of *Who* magazine with two photos of me on the cover (look closely at the photo in the picture gallery). One was the old shot of me in the dress when I was twice my size and the other was the new me, where we had hastily pinned the same dress in to fit my new much smaller chassis. It was a little bit of a hollow victory because as soon as I saw the cover I noticed that in the huge 'after' photo I was showing a bit of nipple, well at least some areola anyway. While the magazine had attempted to airbrush it out, it's a bit like the pimple on your nose that you try desperately to hide with concealer but is still obvious to you.

My rationalisation and reply to all those who also noticed and commented to me about it was that if it was good enough for Elaine in a *Seinfeld* episode to show 'nip' on her Christmas cards, then I guess it was alright for me to show it on the cover of a national magazine.

Then in August 2002, I was overjoyed when *Who* magazine chose me, along with Julia Morris, Sophie Dahl, and Carnie Wilson to grace the cover of their 'Still Half Their Size' issue.

The following year I was approached by Who magazine's life and style editor Simone Casey to be part of a panel of judges critiquing celebrity fashions in their 'Style Council' each week. Depending on the outfit, I'd show my claws or give applause on what they are wearing. Over the next three and a half years I had fun filing my one liners but I was very mindful not to make adverse comments about anyone's size and shape in my comments. I tried to put myself in their shoes each week and think how I'd react if I read the same thing about me.

Unfortunately, my best one liners didn't make it to print.

## Self-first

I often use the term 'self-first' and get asked if there is a difference between being selfish and putting yourself first. My best analogy is when you're on an aircraft and during the safety drill they emphasise that you should put your oxygen mask on first before assisting others.

You also have to learn to find time to put yourself first and that is often the hardest thing to do. Especially if you have a family or have people who are reliant on you. It's imperative that you do certain things for yourself – no-one else!

# Susie's seven ways to strengthen willpower

1 Persistence and determination – focus on the end result!

2 Don't procrastinate, all you're doing is wasting precious time

3 Fail to plan, plan to fail – think ahead to avoid the pitfalls

4 If you fail, don't give up – recognise your downfalls and reassess your approach

5 Don't be a martyr – reward your success but not with food

6 Seek help if you can't find moderation

7 Be honest with yourself

'Success is a journey not a destination – half the fun is getting there.'
– GITA BELLIN

# Timely tips from celebrity lips

**Susie:** What's your best time-management tip?

**Jeff Fenech:** We're losing touch today – kids are in the house playing computers, eating while watching television, and we aren't out doing sport anymore. Computers stop activity, which causes you to put on weight. My tip to anybody is to find some time, just twenty minutes twice a day to do something. If you do something, you always feel much better within yourself. You feel proud and ready for the challenges ahead.

**Fran Macpherson:** Do it. Make lists for everything. If you make a list you'll realise how little you have to do or how much you have to do. But generally you'll find it's less than you think. So, make a list, look at it, be realistic about the list, and cross things off as you go.

**Wayne Pearce:** Time management wise, I think you've got to have a plan for each day. You've got to have the ability to say no. People who don't say no in life tend to get bogged down with things that don't really matter … It's important to prioritise your day … I start off with exercise in the morning, to get it out of the way. By doing this I have no excuses of being too busy with other things.

**Tara Moss:** I think the best time management tip is probably just not to fear things and you'll just get them done.

**Shelley Taylor-Smith:** Procrastination is a waste of time. I just tell people, 'What the heck are you waiting for?' People say, 'I'll wait till I've got more time,' 'I'll wait till it's summer,' 'I'll wait 'till it's winter.' What the heck are you waiting for? Tomorrow could be gone. It's always the right time and the fact that you say you don't have time, means that you aren't being honest with yourself. I've never heard anybody at 80 years of age say, 'I wish I had spent more time in the office.'

**Susie:** We can all make the excuse, particularly with exercise, or eating healthy, that we don't have time. Any preparation tips?

**Sandra Sully:** I am very lucky in Sydney with access to incredible produce, but must stress that healthy options are a matter of choice and planning. There are always healthy options before us, but often through habit and ignorance we just don't see them. We just need to think, give ourselves a minute and not buy on impulse. Make a positive choice instead of a packet of chips.

# CHAPTER 7

# MANAGING THE MENOPAUSE MADNESS

## Weight Gain and Changing Shape

Most women I know can easily tell when their periods are due just by how much, or more likely, how little control they have over their food and chocolate cravings, so I guess since puberty we've known intuitively that hormones and appetite go hand in hand.

My appetite went off the Richter scale going through menopause and I had a terrible time with many menopause symptoms. Some were very hard to contend with, others debilitating, especially the hot flushes and night sweats. My experience though menopause can best be described as horrendous.

It all started when my periods stopped at around 47 years of age, and seemed to continue on and off for another ten years and more. At one point, my night sweats were so bad that I would have to stack piles of towels and cotton T-shirts beside my bed and every hour or two throughout the night I would wake up saturated with sopping wet bed sheets and pillowcases. I'd change my T-shirt and lay fresh towels down and exhaustedly fall back to sleep, only to wake up an hour or two later to do it all again. This went on for months and months on end, night after night after night.

Each morning I'd have to strip the bed and air it all day, wash all the bed linen, towels and T-shirts, then make the bed just before I went to sleep. It was lucky I was single at the time; I'd hate to have put a partner through all that too.

I'm amazed at how much my body shape changed pre, during and after menopause – and not for the better. No matter how much excess weight I've carried on and off throughout my younger life, I always had a defined waistline, but that had filled out.

The change to my body I disliked the most was the thickening of my upper waist between my bust and my belly button. It protruded out in the shape of a turtle shell. At one point, I feared it wouldn't stop swelling and would end up bulging out further than my bust … and believe me that's no mean feat.

My most embarrassing moments during menopause happened when I was live on national TV hosting shows on TVSN, the Shopping Network. To set the scene; like the majority of shows you host on TVSN, this one went for one hour and I was presenting it on my own. The cameras are all robotic and there is no floor manager, so all your instructions come from the control room through your ear piece and the only way you can communicate back to them is verbally but that means everyone watching hears it too.

The only person with me in the studio is a very busy hard-working stage manager, who is bringing in and setting up each new product and product card and taking away the one you've just featured.

On one occasion the camera was on a close-up of my hand when I had an enormous hot flush and suddenly beads of sweat started pouring out of each and every pore and began dripping down my hand and around the jewellery. The crew in the control room were quick to see it happen and switched from a close-up of my hand to a wider mid-shot of me, only to find that the same thing was happening throughout my entire body. You could see I was sweating profusely, as it was running down my face, neck and arms.

The director quickly went to a still photograph of the item I was talking about, so I could grab a bundle of tissues from nearby and quickly mop up my face and hands, while all the time continuing to talk glowingly about the piece of jewellery in front of me. I'm proud to say that I didn't miss a beat. I'm sure very few people watching would have known what I was going through. My hot flushes happened several times more throughout that live television show, which, at the time, felt like it was going for much longer than its scheduled hour.

The hot flushes continued relentlessly during many other live TV shows after that, but we soon worked out a signal that I could give to the crew in the control room, whenever I could feel another hot flush coming on, so they could quickly go to other vision each time I needed to mop up the flood of perspiration.

You'd think with me losing what felt like bucketloads of sweat each day and night that I'd have lost weight in the process … sadly, no!

# Dr Gary Aaron interview

I found I wasn't alone when it came to the insatiable appetite, the weight gain, the thickening waist line, and other changes in my shape. Other women I know in perimenopause and menopause have shared similar experiences and symptoms so I thought it was important to find out why all this happens and to see if there is anything we can do to reduce or prevent these negative menopause changes to our body from occurring.

I knew the best person to ask would be Dr Gary Aaron MB BCh, FAARM, Dip. Acup.

Dr Gary is CEO and medical director of Australian Menopause Centre (AMC), overseeing a team of over 40 staff including doctors, specialised clinical staff and naturopaths. He's a member of the American Academy of Anti-Aging Medicine, has completed his fellowship in Anti-Ageing and Regenerative Medicine and is now a Fellow of the American Academy of Anti-Ageing Medicine and is Board Certified.

The Australian Menopause Centre's treatment program is comprehensive and includes access to bio-identical hormones, also known as body-identical hormones, derived from plants (Mexican wild yams). As I understand it, they have exactly the same chemical and molecular structure as the hormones that are produced by our body. I was pleased recently to see that the medical profession is now endorsing much of what Dr Gary's been adopting in his practice for decades.

While Dr Gary wasn't around to help me through my menopause nightmare, I've interviewed him extensively since on my talkback radio show. Dr Gary's extensive knowledge and ability to explain complex medical terms and conditions simply and easily, made him very popular with my radio listeners and I'm delighted he's agreed to share his expertise in this book.

Dr Gary is passionate about anti-aging in both men and women and after spending time with him and his impressive AMC team I didn't hesitate to accept his invitation to be the Ambassador for the Australian Menopause Centre (AMC).

As part of their holistic and natural approach to good health and anti-ageing a huge focus at the AMC is on diet and lifestyle. The role their team of naturopaths and specialised clinical staff play is to identify and remove the barriers to good health. They also provide weight loss and healthy eating guidelines to help create the ideal food fuel to keep our dream car running at optimal and be our dream car size and shape.

**Susie:** Dr Gary Aaron why do our hormone fluctuations over 28 days directly impact on women's appetites?

**Dr Gary Aaron:** What we know is that during a woman's reproductive years, her hormones go through a regular cycle each month. During the second half of her cycle, her oestrogen levels climb progressively over the two weeks leading up to her period. Normally, the body will produce enough progesterone to balance this oestrogen build up. In some women, the oestrogen production is excessive during these two weeks or the progesterone production is insufficient. This imbalance of a high oestrogen to progesterone ratio is what stimulates sweet cravings. This can be quite an extreme craving and of course promotes significant weight gain.

**Susie:** What is menopause?

**Dr Gary Aaron:** By definition, menopause is the pausing of the menses, the end of a woman's menstrual periods. However, clinically it doesn't make sense to define it as a point in time when the menses stop. I break down these changes into three stages: perimenopause, menopause proper, and post menopause. They are each distinguished by their symptoms which reflect the hormone changes that are occurring.

Perimenopause occurs when ovulation ceases or becomes erratic. This results in a lower production of progesterone during the second half of the cycle – referred to as the luteal phase. As the oestrogen concentration increases the progesterone production is not keeping up. An imbalance between the oestrogen and progesterone, results in the classic symptoms of fluid retention, breast tenderness, weight gain, irritability, headaches, and sleeplessness.

In menopause proper, the production of oestrogen slows down throughout the cycle. Menopausal women have a combined oestrogen and progesterone deficiency. The most common symptoms of menopause include hot flushes, night sweats, dry skin, vaginal dryness, feeling emotional, feeling fatigued, poor memory as well as a low libido.

Once a woman becomes post-menopausal, she is no longer feeling the effects of her low hormones to the same degree. Her hot flushes and night sweats settle, her moods lift, her energy improves. Often some of the menopause symptoms remain, particularly the vaginal dryness and low libido, but mostly the symptoms do not disrupt her life significantly.

**Susie:** Why do some women suffer and others seem to breeze through menopause?

**Dr Gary Aaron:** In my practice, I recognise three groups of women going through these hormone changes:

1. Those that have severe symptoms of perimenopause; a mild menopause often follows this.
2. Those that have very few perimenopause symptoms; they drop heavily into menopause and suffer significantly from oestrogen progesterone deficiency.
3. Those that have very mild symptoms of both oestrogen and progesterone symptoms.

I have not come across any literature that explains this third phenomenon but an explanation of the first two groups may shed some light.

The women who experience severe symptoms of perimenopause are often more sensitive to the presence of oestrogen. I refer to them as 'oestrogen dominant'. The cell receptors that are specific for oestrogen are overly sensitive, resulting in an overreaction to oestrogen. Progesterone competes with oestrogen for these receptors and will block or dampen the effect of oestrogen on the receptors. So, when progesterone declines, this oestrogen dominance becomes more significant. The receptors respond even to a very low level of oestrogen so these women are less likely to experience symptoms of oestrogen deficiency.

Women who have severe symptoms of menopause have oestrogen and progesterone receptors with a 'normal' degree of sensitivity. Once the levels of these hormones decline, the individual experiences the absolute deficiency of these hormones – there is no back-up from sensitive oestrogen receptors.

Theoretically, those women who don't experience symptoms of menopause or perimenopause, will likely have cell receptors that are hypersensitive to both oestrogen and progesterone, so even when the hormone levels are low, the cell receptors are still able to transmit a message to the cell, avoiding the symptoms of deficiency. So, these women will remain symptom free throughout the process of the 'change of life'.

**Susie:** What causes the hot flushes, night sweats, mood swings, hair thinning, loss of libido and all the other terrible symptoms?

**Dr Gary Aaron:** Mostly, each symptom reflects a deficiency or an excess of one or other hormone. This may vary from person to person however the symptoms below most commonly reflect the hormone deficiency/excess listed:

| | |
|---|---|
| Hot flushes | Oestrogen deficiency |
| Night sweats | Oestrogen deficiency |
| Night time overheating | Oestrogen excess and/or progesterone deficiency |
| Mood swings | Oestrogen excess and/or progesterone deficiency |
| Feeling emotional | Oestrogen excess and/or progesterone deficiency |
| Breast tenderness | Oestrogen excess and/or progesterone deficiency |
| Fluid retention | Oestrogen excess and/or progesterone deficiency |
| Weight gain | Oestrogen excess and/or progesterone deficiency |
| Break through bleeding | Oestrogen excess and/or progesterone deficiency |
| Headaches | Oestrogen build up or an oestrogen drop off |
| Sleeplessness | Oestrogen excess and/or progesterone deficiency |
| Low libido | Low testosterone, low oestrogen |
| Hair loss/thinning | Low progesterone, testosterone excess |

**Susie:** Why can't we just simply take more oestrogen?

**Dr Gary Aaron:** As described above, each woman presents differently with different causes for her symptom complex. By giving oestrogen to a woman who is oestrogen sensitive – oestrogen dominant – you are feeding fuel to the flame. Oestrogen given to an oestrogen dominant person will promote weight gain, breast tenderness, breakthrough bleeding and headaches.

A vital understanding that many medical practitioners don't have is that we cannot treat all women with a one-size-fits-all treatment. Each woman's needs are highly specific and these needs do change over the course of her transition. Treatment needs to be based on a woman's needs for that time of her perimenopause/menopause.

**Susie:** Why do you keep your menopause treatment as natural as possible?

**Dr Gary Aaron:** Bio-identical Hormone Replacement Therapy (BHRT) used to be called natural HRT. The term 'natural' has three meanings for me:

1. The active ingredients are extracted from wild yam. There are no non-plant active ingredients in BHRT.
2. The biochemical structure of the hormones used in BHRT – the oestrogen, progesterone and testosterone – all have a biochemical structure that is identical to what the patient is producing herself. This is distinct from most synthetic HRT products like Premarin and Provera that have a chemical structure considerably different to what the body produces naturally.
3. BHRT is compounded on a patient-by-patient basis. This allows for the correct combination of hormones for each individual. This is different to the commercial products where it is a one-size-fits-all treatment.

The combination of these three factors is why I prefer to prescribe BHRT specific for each individual's needs, rather than a one-size-fits-all treatment.

**Susie:** Why does menopause have such an impact on our metabolism causing weight gain, fat storage, and big changes to our body shape?

**Dr Gary Aaron:** Our body relies on the correct balance of our hormones for normal function. If one or more hormones decline, as occurs in perimenopause and/or menopause, it impacts our normal functioning as well as our metabolism.

The most significant impact on weight gain around this stage is the impact of oestrogen dominance. Oestrogen has an effect of retaining fluid in our body tissues. Progesterone on the other hand, works like a natural diuretic. When the progesterone drops or the oestrogen climbs, the net effect is fluid retention and weight gain. Most fluid retention due to oestrogen occurs in the breasts and around the waist. So, the shape change that occurs in women with oestrogen dominance is a move from the pear shape to the apple shape.

**Susie:** Why do you place such a strong focus on diet and lifestyle at AMC?

**Dr Gary Aaron:** As we age and our hormones decline, we are exposed to many medical conditions that if considered early, can be avoided. The most important conditions that are avoidable are osteoporosis and diabetes. Osteoporosis occurs due to a deficiency of calcium in the bone. It predisposes to fractures. There are two major things happening that cause osteoporosis:

1.  Insufficient calcium deposition into the bone – not enough osteoblast activity or bone growth; and
2.  Excessive breakdown of bone and loss of calcium – too much osteoclastic activity and demineralisation.

Besides ensuring an adequate intake of calcium in the diet, weight-bearing exercises can prove very helpful in preventing or even reversing osteoporosis.

With diabetes, our diet is important in preventing insulin resistance and rising glucose levels. This can be controlled by a strong focus on diet and exercise.

**Susie:** Are there foods we should avoid that intensify menopause symptoms?

**Dr Gary Aaron:** The major impact of some foods is to intensify some of the symptoms – particularly hot flushes and night sweats. Many patients have reported how hot and spicy foods can worsen their symptoms. In other patients, alcohol can often bring on their symptoms. Each patient reacts differently to certain foods. If you know that a particular food or liquid brings on symptoms, then it's best to avoid those specific foods.

**Susie:** Are there any foods to include in our food fuel that will prevent or reduce the symptoms of menopause?

**Dr Gary Aaron:** I don't generally advocate avoiding any specific foods unless the individual knows that she reacts negatively to something. However, I do advocate a healthy diet – high in fruit and vegetables, good fats, and protein, and avoid as much as possible, simple carbohydrates like sugar, pastas, potatoes, sweets, confectionery etcetera.

**Susie:** Do men go through menopause too?

**Dr Gary Aaron:** Yes, men experience a more gradual decline in their major sex hormone – testosterone. Men's testosterone levels peak in their late teenage years. There is a gradual decline thereafter of approximately 1–2 per cent per year for the rest of their life. As such, the onset of symptoms is more subtle and feels more like a gradual ageing process rather than a sudden onset of severe symptoms.

**Susie:** What are their symptoms? What can men do to stop or help reduce these symptoms?

**Dr Gary Aaron:** Symptoms most commonly felt by men experiencing testosterone insufficiency or deficiency include the following:

- Low energy
- Low libido
- Muscle wasting
- Moodiness – described as a 'bear with a sore head'
- Erectile dysfunction
- Night sweats
- Poor concentration and low motivation

Stress can bring on andropause (male menopause) a lot quicker so developing techniques to control and deal with stress is important. Exercise and a healthy diet, reduce alcohol intake and cut down or quit smoking would be the major ways to improve or reduce symptoms of testosterone deficiency.

**Susie:** Carrying visceral fat around our waist not only feels and looks uncomfortable but it is very dangerous for our internal health, isn't it?

**Dr Gary Aaron:** Abdominal obesity or an increase in waist circumference is a well-recognised predictor of risk for conditions like heart disease, cancer, or other causes of mortality in middle-aged women. The most notable study done relating abdominal obesity to risk is called the Nurses' Health study.

**Susie:** What causes a 'beer belly' in men and what does it take to get rid of it?

**Dr Gary Aaron:** The term 'beer belly' is a colloquialism used to refer to central obesity and to those people who have it. Even though it is common in beer drinkers, there is little evidence that beer drinkers are more prone to central obesity. It is equally common in non-drinkers and wine and spirits drinkers. The major cause of central obesity is net energy balance – there are more calories being consumed than are being expended. Other conditions such as insulin resistance can contribute to this imbalance.

In simple terms, to lose weight, energy expenditure should be greater than energy intake. So, a good and consistent exercise regime together with limiting the amount of food intake and improving the kind of foods consumed will help to get rid of the 'beer belly'.

**Susie:** What are your top three tips to avoid gaining weight during menopause?

**Dr Gary Aaron:** The hardest condition to counteract is oestrogen dominance, simply because it is out of one's control. Women who lack progesterone or who are hypersensitive to oestrogen will often have controlled healthy diets and strong exercise regimes but will still be gaining weight.

Tip 1: If you suspect oestrogen dominance, either introduce progesterone or an alternative treatment to balance your hormone levels.

Tip 2: Diet is not just what you eat but more importantly, how much you eat. Your food choices should include a colourful selection of fruit and vegetables, lots of protein and good fats and limited simple carbohydrates. Your volume of food intake can be helped by using a few varied ideas:

- Eat off a side plate rather than a normal plate – it reduces the surface area to half.
- Time yourself at each meal – it should take you no less than 20 minutes to finish what's on your plate. You will be surprised how this can help you reach satiety without overeating.
- Drink lots of water each day – minimum 2 litres but more like 3 or 4 litres.
- Chew your food for longer
- Use small cutlery – it works!

# CHAPTER 8

# TWENTY-FIRST CENTURY DISCOVERIES

## 'Fat Virus' – Is Obesity Contagious?

The 'fat virus' sounds like an excuse equivalent to 'the dog ate my homework' and a foodaholic's dream come true, but it seems there is such a thing.

Richard Atkinson MD, Emeritus Professor of Medicine and Nutrition at the University of Wisconsin describes it as an adenovirus called Ad36 and according to his research, it may account for some 30 per cent of the world's obesity problems. Professor Atkinson has led several investigations of Ad36 with studies involving animals and humans. The virus was given to mice, rats, chickens and monkeys and published studies have shown their body fat increases by 50–100 per cent despite being fed the same amount as animals not given the virus. Professor Atkinson believes the virus seems to change body composition, so there is an increased percentage of fat, and the monkey gained about four times more weight than the virus-free comparison monkeys.

He also presented data at two scientific conferences on a study that will soon appear in an issue of the *International Journal of Obesity*. This study was conducted in three US cities involving more than 500 obese and healthy-weight people who had their blood tested for antibodies to the Ad36 virus. The results showed around 30 per cent of obese people had antibodies to the Ad36 virus and were quite significantly heavier, compared to just 10 per cent of healthy-weight people. If these results are true then the Ad36 virus could be a contributing factor to our worldwide epidemic of obesity and why we are seeing obesity levels rising at extremely high levels outside the First World countries.

## Could stress be making us fat?

In 2014 scientists at the Monash University School of Biomedical Sciences discovered the stress hormone cortisol could be a reason why some people gain weight over others, and find it harder to lose it. The research found low cortisol responders were more likely to eat less and showed an increase in physical activity. High cortisol responders, with a predisposition to obesity, didn't reduce their food intake in response to stress and burnt fewer kilojoules. The study further revealed the different metabolic responses and behaviours to stress. Forty volunteers have been recruited for human trials by Monash University, headed up by Dr Kevin Lee, Professor Iain Clarke and Dr Belinda Henry, and I'll be very keen to see the results.

## Fibre and good gut health

This book isn't only viewing our food fuel through a weight-management prism. Through extensive research, twenty-first century thinking now puts fibre on a pedestal as being critical to good gut health. Fibre may also help you age well and possibly even lengthen your life.

I'm constantly reading about systemic inflammation playing a key role in our bodies getting sick and developing major diseases and fibre could be the 'knight in shining armour' to the rescue.

To find out more I've called upon Dr Maxwell Strong PhD, founder of the Institute of Aging & Clinical Nutrition Inc, who's been a medical researcher for several decades and a consultant to a number of major international pharmaceutical, food and beverage companies. Since the late 2000s Dr Strong's principal research has involved working with dietary fibre. As the Chief Scientist and CEO of Neurolex Pty Ltd, he's developed a drug-free soluble 100 per cent vegetable prebiotic fibre known as Neurolex.

# Dr Maxwell Strong interview

**Susie:** What is fibre?

**Dr Maxwell Strong:** Dietary fibre, sometimes called roughage, is the indigestible part of the foods we eat and in a healthy diet the chief sources are fruits and vegetables, cereals and whole grains.

**Susie:** Do we need to eat specific fibre? What about the fibre that's currently in our diet?

**Dr Maxwell Strong:** Fibre in our diet is usually categorised as either soluble or insoluble fibre and we need a regular intake of both for healthy function. The problem is that the large majority of us consume a 'Western diet' which characteristically is high in fats, refined carbohydrates such as sucrose, and low in fibre. In fact most of us consume less than half the recommended daily intake of fibre.

**Susie:** What foods and lifestyle choices contribute to poor gut health and cause systemic inflammation?

**Dr Maxwell Strong:** Most of our major age-related causes of premature morbidity and mortality in industrialised countries have a lifestyle component as a key component in their initiation and progression. These might include smoking and excess alcohol intake, excess energy (calorie) intake, poor diet, and lack of regular activity such as walking etcetera. These choices, along with the ageing process itself, lead to intestinal dysbiosis or an excess of toxic or pathogenic resident gut microbes over those which are known to be health-promoting.

**Susie:** What has your research and the data you've drawn from numerous studies in Australia and overseas shown about the benefits of eating soluble fibre?

**Dr Maxwell Strong:** Most published university epidemiological studies demonstrate that populations with diets which are habitually high in certain types of fibre are characterised by lower rates of many chronic diseases. A recent Sydney University published study is such an example. This study followed the diets of 1600 adults for a period of ten years and found that those participants whose diets were highest in what was categorised as 'indigestible' fibre had an 80 per cent likelihood of ageing longer, disease-free and fully-functional than those with the lowest intake of this fibre.

Our research for more than a decade has shown that the key to healthy ageing and longevity found with this type of 'indigestible fibre' is that it passes undigested to the large intestine where it is metabolised by particular families of resident bacteria, producing short-chain fatty acids, particularly butyrate, as metabolites. And it's this amazing gut-produced natural chemical, butyrate, which is demonstrated in an ever-increasing body of robust published science to be responsible for this health-promoting effect.

**Susie:** What is a prebiotic? I understand soluble fibre works best when taken as a prebiotic.

**Dr Maxwell Strong:** A prebiotic fibre is the term used for that fibre which passes undigested to the large intestine where it very selectively feeds only the health-promoting bacteria as described above, correcting the condition of dysbiosis, common to many of us.

**Susie:** You're now a self-confessed very active, youthful great-grandfather and octogenarian, who has survived three major medically documented life-threatening events including sudden cardiac death, aggressive inoperable cancer and ischemic stroke. Please share your concept of building a protective cognitive reserve?

**Dr Maxwell Strong:** Two of our major causes of morbidity and mortality, stroke and Alzheimer's disease, are the result of trauma to the brain, the former being the result of an acute trauma and the second a chronic trauma taking place with loss of brain cells and connections (synapses) over a long period of time, even perhaps decades, but both sharing a common loss of brain cells.

It is now clear in our research that the best defence against these two disastrous major diseases is in building an adequate brain cognitive reserve and plasticity resulting from butyrate-induced BDNF brain levels, and which allows the brain to adjust to correct and successfully survive this brain trauma.

The fact that this fibre has been a key component in my diet during the last seven years, building a high level of brain cognitive reserve, has allowed me to so successfully survive the trauma of an ischemic stroke.

**Susie:** Why did you choose chicory root as the 100 per cent soluble vegetable fibre in the prebiotic you've developed?

**Dr Maxwell Strong:** Optimising the butyrate yields of this vegetable tuber fibre has been a key area of our research, resulting in a low-cost, soluble fibre which can be conveniently added daily to a range of foods and beverages including tea and coffee, juices or water.

**Susie:** Do we need to make this a lifestyle change and add soluble fibre to our food fuel mix daily?

**Dr Maxwell Strong:** I am constantly reminded that I am the best advertisement of the success of habitual use of this soluble, indigestible dietary fibre, and I am now joined by an ever-increasing group of enthusiastic Neurolex ambassadors attesting to the health-promoting effects of this safe, drug-free natural fibre.

To read the scientific research into the benefits of eating soluble fibre or to contact Dr Maxwell Strong go to Neurolex.com.au.

## Dieting ages your face

I've always felt I looked older when carrying excess weight but it now seems that the opposite could be true. A US research study carried out on 200 pairs of identical twins compared their appearance and BMI (which is calculated by dividing your weight by your height times two). The survey concluded that losing the equivalent of one dress size can age women by four years. Women with plumper cheeks were found to look younger than slimmer women. Dieting was found to be up there with divorce, depression, sunbathing, smoking and drinking as a major factor in making women look older.

According to Senior Researcher Dr Bahaman Guyuron, A BMI higher by four points was found to result in a younger appearance of between two and four years in women over 40 years old.

That doesn't mean we should ditch the healthy lifestyle changes and pile on the pounds just to keep a more youthful face. Now that I'm Still Half My Size I'm in much better health than when I was carrying 50 plus kilograms more. I find people now tell me that I look younger and I certainly feel younger.

A good mate of mine Mandy, who's been in the beauty business for decades, often jokes that the easiest way to look younger and slimmer is to hang around with people who are older and fatter than you!

## Free Get Healthy Service

In 2010, I was invited to take part in a study with around 800 participants conducted by the School of Public Health at the University of Sydney, in collaboration with the New South Wales Department of Health. We were enrolled in the NSW Get Healthy Information and Coaching Service.

It's a free telephone and web-based service and involved getting lots of very helpful information beforehand about healthy eating and physical activity, then receiving regular phone calls from qualified health coaches to monitor our progress and help us reach and maintain a healthy weight. It's since been successfully expanded to most states. Put Get Healthy into your internet search engine to see if this free service is available where you live or call 1300 806 258 or visit GetHealthyNSW.com.au.

# CHAPTER 9

# SECRETS FROM THE STARS

Fran Macpherson interview

E
ver wondered what Elle Macpherson's mum fed her to help her grow up to be a supermodel? When I first meet Fran Macpherson I could immediately see where all her children inherited their good looks, but as I spent more time with her I also learnt how disciplined she is with her eating and exercise.

Fran Macpherson has been living low-fat just about her entire life. Fran understands better than most about body image and how much harder it gets, the older you get. I was chatting with her on the phone one night as she was preparing for a dinner party, where everything she served was 'unleaded' but none of her guests knew. Fran's a terrific cook so it all tasted yummy. Some of her great low-fat recipes are in the back of this book including a couple of great low-fat soups. In the interview that follows Fran gives lots of sensible eating tips that she gave to all her children: Elle, Mimi, Ben and Lissie.

**Susie:** Please tell me the Fran Macpherson story.

**Macpherson:** I was born in Brisbane, moved to Sydney in the early 1950s. We lived in Manly, the family came to Sydney because Dad had sold his business in Brisbane and he wanted to open a cafe. Never did open the cafe. He went into real estate. I started nursing at Royal North Shore Hospital and I went to a party at Sydney Uni when I was about nine months into my nursing career. At that party I met my first husband. I was very naive. That was a chequered relationship, which resulted in my three eldest children.

We separated after about nine years and then I met and married Neill Macpherson. We had a child in 1982: that's my baby Elizabeth. We all went to live in Asia in 1983 and came back to Australia 1992, when our marriage broke up.

**Susie:** Were you a fussy eater as a child?

**Macpherson:** Heavens no! The only thing I refused to eat was rice pudding, mashed potato with lumps, offal, except tripe and brains. I was a bit of a pig, I was chubby.

**Susie:** Were you?

**Macpherson:** I was chubby. I went to a friend's farm for the school holidays when I was about twelve, when I came back I was like a balloon blown up. My mother barely recognised her little blue-eyed, blonde twelve-year-old. I remember not being able to fit into my pink jeans. I loved those pink jeans more than anything.

**Susie:** Were you good at sport?

**Macpherson:** I'm a sporty person. Swimmer, runner, netball player.

**Susie:** You are tall, but do you still have to watch your weight?

**Macpherson:** Constantly! It's called living your life on a diet. But now I do it without thinking, so it's not living my life on a diet. If I pick at someone's chips, I don't think about it anymore. Once upon a time I would have bashed myself up over it. I exercise a lot, not as much as I should for my age group, but I do exercise quite a bit. I am very, very careful with what I eat. I've totally cut some things from my diet.

**Susie:** Let's run through some of the things that you've totally eliminated.

**Macpherson:** I only eat the fat that I don't know I'm eating, as in when I go to a restaurant. Even though I try to stick to the grilled fish and salad or vegies, sometimes I get seduced by delicious-sounding choices. I never have butter or any other spread. I don't like the taste of fat anymore. I couldn't eat ice-cream – I love it but I don't do it, or cream or custard. Full-cream milk changes the taste of my morning tea; I haven't had full cream milk for so long. I now use absolutely no fat milk, which is fine, because it's still got calcium content and I like the taste.

I'm not absolutely vegetarian, I do eat meat although not that often. I eat chicken sometimes, lots and lots of fish, lots of vegetables and fruit and enough nuts to complement my diet. When I want to nibble at something I nibble at almonds and dates; I love dates – must be the sugar, so I try not to eat too many but they are my treat.

**Susie:** So what do you eat for breakfast, for instance?

**Macpherson:** The same thing almost every day of my life (laughs). A piece of fruit, a cup of tea, and one or two slices of a heavy soy bread, toasted, with vegemite and tomato. It is yummy. If I go out for breakfast it's a treat and I have my eggs. Normally I get up early and run. I take my fruit and eat it on the way to the park or I'll eat it between my apartment building and the corner (laughs).

**Susie:** How often do you do that?

**Macpherson:** Most days of the week. Not on weekends. I try to do it five days a week. Sometimes it can only be four, depending on how early I have to schedule meetings. You have to remember I opt to exercise every moment I can, so I walk up steps, I will walk up my apartment stairs and walk down my stairs. I live in Darlinghurst so I walk everywhere. I always walk to the city or Edgecliff; for me, it's a pleasure.

**Susie:** What about lunch?

**Macpherson:** I rarely have it. My body works better on two meals a day. If I eat lunch, I won't eat dinner. I don't need dinner. I had a very big lunch today and I won't even start feeling hungry until tomorrow morning. That's how my body works, it may not be right, and others may say it's not good for you, but it's how my body operates. I think my body slows down because it knows how much food intake it gets a day.

When I do eat dinner, if I am on my own I will have vegetable-based meals. I do a big vegetable bake and eat it, I love soup and at the moment I am having lots of broccoli and cauliflower, Asian greens and tofu. Chicken stock is always in my pantry for making soup. Also tomato paste: I like using tinned tomatoes when I make ratatouille. I eat a lot of tuna, lots of raw fish. I eat at least one large raw-fish meal a week and then I might have two or three other fish meals a week.

**Susie:** What about pasta, rice, bread …?

**Macpherson:** Love pasta. Love rice. But I rarely eat pasta. I think pasta hangs around in your body for too long and for that reason I eat very little of it, although they say it is good for us. I make a really great 99 per cent fat-free noodle soup, which I love and I might have that a couple of nights a week. I compensate for pasta. I prefer heavy soy bread that I slice myself – tastes better and fills me up more.

**Susie:** What about your pig-out food? Do you eat chocolate?

**Macpherson:** I bought so much chocolate for my kids at Easter, the fridge was full with wonderful eggs. After Easter I put all the eggs and the bunnies that were left over into the freezer with one of those huge Toblerone bars that I had been given. Usually I'm not tempted by chocolate. But I started eating the leftover Easter chocolate and I had to finish that chocolate. I ate the lot. I ate the bunnies, the Toblerone, the eggs, everything. But that's the only time I've pigged out on chocolates for years and years. My downfall is if anyone is eating chips, hot chips, I will pick at them from other people's plates. Terrible manners, but they are so tempting – of course, we all know they don't put on weight because you haven't ordered them!

**Susie:** What about alcohol?

**Macpherson:** Love it. I try really hard to have two nights a week without any alcohol. Two nights is normal, three nights I aspire to, four nights I'm so proud of myself.

**Susie:** What do you think makes you fat?

**Macpherson:** In my case, lack of exercise is the most important thing. I'm not talking generally, everyone is different. I don't consider I overeat, maybe at times I need to eat more, because my metabolism slows down, particularly in the afternoon when it's slowing down because I haven't had any food since maybe 8 am. So I really am conscious that I don't eat enough to keep my metabolism going.

**Susie:** Do you have coffee much through the day?

**Macpherson:** One cup of coffee a day, not every day, but during the week I do. I sometimes go to my favourite coffee shop on the weekend as I love my coffee and newspaper. I prefer to buy a good cappuccino than make myself an ordinary coffee. If I am going to drink it, it has to be good.

**Susie:** Do you think fat makes you fat?

**Macpherson:** No, I think every time you open your mouth and put something in it that you shouldn't, it makes you fat. I am a believer that all food that you put in your mouth should be beneficial. That's what I believe, what I do is another thing. What makes you fat? Too much of anything makes you fat, a little bit makes you happy.

**Susie:** Is running your first preference for exercise?

**Macpherson:** Yes. I loathe the gym.

**Susie:** So, what happens if it's raining?

**Macpherson:** Look last night, I went to bed and said, 'Please rain, please rain, I don't want to get up.' It didn't rain. So I had to get up. If it's raining I have a wonderful time with my tea and a book or sometimes I dance around the house. I put on some music and dance for an hour. I love that because no-one is watching me.

**Susie:** Now, you've got some great recipes that you are going to give us for the book.

**Macpherson:** I sure am.

**Susie:** Who taught you and what's your favourite recipe?

**Macpherson:** Growing up with a mother who was such a good cook and she was different, she wasn't traditional. She used to say we are what we eat. So I was lucky to grow up with a woman who considered that what you put into your body showed.

She said 'Put starving children in front of a table full of food and they will first go to what the body needs.' I think listen to your body is probably one of the most important things. What does your body tell you? My body tells me that meat makes me feel sluggish, meat makes me not sleep very well, meat tastes good once a month, my body needs it then. Vegetables make me happy, they make me smile and they make me go yum yum. Maybe that's extreme, but I can go yum yum over a plate of vegies, I promise. (laughs)

**Susie:** If you're entertaining, which you do regularly, will you alter things in any way? Or will you still feed your guests the same low-fat way you live?

**Macpherson:** Everyone gets low-fat, they don't know it's low-fat, well I don't think they do, because I never think it tastes low-fat. For instance, I make tarts, which certainly aren't low-fat, as you've got pastry. I make my own pesto so there's less oil in it, but there will be pine nuts, which are good for you. But no, they'll eat the same low-fat food.

**Susie:** Does it get harder or easier as you get older?

**Macpherson:** Easier. Because I don't think about it, there is nothing to think about, this is how I live.

**Susie:** So technically, you're not on a diet. You've altered your lifestyle to the way you want to live.

**Macpherson:** If you look at the French word for diet it's regime. It's a regime of living: how we eat our food, what we do. The word diet in our language, English, does have the connotations of deprivation and it's not the real meaning of diet.

**Susie:** You and your children attended the Australasian premiere of *Batman Forever* some years ago and there were lots of comments that you looked more like you were Elle's sister than her mother.

**Macpherson:** Really? Lucky genes. I came from a lucky gene family. I don't know what to say. I abuse myself: I smoke, I drink but I am very careful about what I eat, and I love not being fat, because I thought I was a fat kid. It's a terrible stigma to be a fat kid. I was pregnant at sixteen, had my first child at seventeen. I was a fat teenager. Only after my son did I start to look at my diet and lifestyle in some conscious way – and I haven't stopped doing that since.

**Susie:** Given that your mother obviously set you up with a good eating education, what approach to food and exercise did you take with your children when they were growing up?

**Macpherson:** If you ask any of those kids, they'll tell you that I starved them as children! Mimi will say she lived on the Atkins diet and that's why she's so skinny. The fact is she takes after her father who is very skinny. Brendan, my son, used to walk around saying 'Mum if you don't give me meat, I'm going to fade away.' Of course Bren's six foot two.

I don't come from the 'you must eat everything' family. The starving children of China aren't going to get my scraps. I didn't want my children to feel that food is a punishment or a treat. If they didn't want to eat it then I didn't make them eat it, but there were no substitutes – eat what you were given or nothing. Really hard but necessary in a big family. At that point, I was starting to explore the theory of if your body needed it, it would be eaten, if your body didn't need it then it was overindulgence.

**Susie:** So you wouldn't give them something sweeter or were there treats in place of it?

**Macpherson:** Very few treats in our house. Still not. But we'd have big birthday parties and I used to make cakes and cookies and things. The cakes were generally pound cakes, which the other kids didn't like much though – but my kids did!

**Susie:** Did you ever let your kids have those sort of fast foods and all that?

**Macpherson:** I'm a cheat of a mother. I'm full of all this great advice, I loved my kids having McDonald's. You have to understand, McDonald's is fine for kids as long as it's in moderation. I used to watch my sister forbidding her boys in London to have McDonald's, I would say 'you're crazy, it's like forbidding them to drink alcohol, they're going to race out and do it behind your back.' You do not forbid anybody to do anything.

**Susie:** How do you stay in shape with a jet-setting lifestyle? If you are not working here, you're off visiting family somewhere in the world.

**Macpherson:** I guess the lucky gene pool fits in there a bit. Also remember that I do find time to exercise, so if it's running in the park or dancing at home, I try to do something. I can spend an hour with the music on, it may not be hugely aerobic, but it's getting the blood moving, flicking the legs and arms, it's movement.

# Wayne Pearce interview

I've never met anyone more dedicated than football legend Wayne Pearce when it comes to what fuel he puts into his body and how he burns it off. Wayne's leadership and team-building skills are widely acknowledged in the sporting community. He not only captained the highly successful Balmain Tigers club for eight seasons (1983–90), but also led the New South Wales State of Origin side in ten games.

In 1994 he turned his hand to coaching the then lowly placed Tigers and before long he moulded them into a tightknit and highly competitive outfit. His outstanding efforts saw him appointed as New South Wales State of Origin coach in 1999 and in the 2000 season he became the only person to both captain and coach a series whitewash (3–0 victory).

Wayne left club coaching in September 2000 to focus his energy on corporate team-building and personal-development programs. I got to know a bit about Wayne's past, when he joined a number of other national celebrities to take part in the Keep Our Kids Alive Drug Awareness weekend in Port Macquarie. Wayne has amazing willpower and is the closest example I know of someone living the 'text book' healthy lifestyle.

**Susie:** What made Wayne Pearce?

**Wayne Pearce:** I was born and raised inner-city in Balmain, to very much working-class, blue-collar parents. My father worked on the council as a street sweeper and my mother was an office secretary at the Colgate Palmolive factory, which was in Balmain at the time.

I went to the local primary school; there were about 90 kids in the whole school. Even after starting high school I really didn't have much of an idea about what to achieve in life. I just bumbled along until my father died suddenly and unexpectedly in Sydney when I was fourteen while Mum, my two brothers and I were away on a holiday in western New South Wales. That was a major turning point in my life.

Dad had three brothers who all died from cardiovascular disease before they reached 50, so they were quite young. When the anger and grief subsided I started to do some thinking and thought about the fact that he drank a lot, and smoked a lot, and didn't eat the right foods, so I thought, well, I'd better start looking after myself. For some strange reason, something clicked in my head that I wanted to prove myself, so I started to apply myself to footy and in the process of that I thought I wanted to know more about how you can be fitter and healthier.

To cut a long story short, rather than just doing the School Certificate I set myself new goals: to go to year twelve and also do university – which none of my family had ever done. I completed a Science degree, and also a Dip Ed, with three years psychology as part of the Science degree as well. If my father hadn't died in the manner he did, I probably wouldn't have developed the motivation to sting me out of the slumber I was in.

**Susie:** As a child how was your diet?

**Wayne Pearce:** I've got plenty of fillings to prove that I ate too many lollies and sweet things as a kid even though I used to clean my teeth regularly. I ate whatever there was to eat. In fact, I ate a lot of junk food as well. Unfortunately junk food was cheap so because we didn't have that much money, I ate a fair bit of cheap junk food. It wasn't until my father died that I started to go down the track of health and fitness. When I first started playing rugby league I arrived with a bit of a reputation as a health and fitness freak. I was definitely not like that as a kid.

**Susie:** Mentally, were there ever times that you felt like giving up?

**Wayne Pearce:** I never felt like giving up. The darkest hour for me was when Dad died and I didn't have a chance to say goodbye. Because we had no money, and me being the eldest of us three boys, my main thought was, 'What can I do here to help us go forward?' At times there was a sense of hopelessness and confusion, but I never felt like giving up. I had this nervous energy and wanted to channel it in the right way; there was an indecisiveness as to which direction was the right way, but never did I think about really giving up.

**Susie:** Do you have to watch your weight?

**Wayne Pearce:** No, I don't. For twenty years my weight has varied by one or two kilos either way of what I am. I think different people require different amounts of nutrients. There are some guys that I played with who are much heavier than me and eat much less than me, but carry a lot of weight. I think that just their base metabolic rate is a lot lower and a lot of that is to do with genetics. People are different. So you shouldn't really judge what you eat against the person alongside of you.

**Susie:** So what do you think makes a person fat?

**Wayne Pearce:** I think it's their frame of mind. Many of us lie to ourselves on a regular basis and in so many ways. And I am talking not just in regards to food but also how we look, what we are capable of achieving, and as a result of that we never quite fulfil our dreams. We have the capacity to design our own lives, but so many of us don't want to assume that responsibility and don't understand that in the palm of our hand, we control our future.

**Susie:** What is glycaemic index or GI?

**Wayne Pearce:** It's simply a measure of the rate of use of the sugars in a food. Sugars that are metabolised quickly are called high GI; sugars that are metabolised more slowly are called low GI.

I think it's important to understand that there are a lot of professional athletes who now understand that fluctuating blood-sugar levels lead us to bingeing on particular foods. I mean if we eat a bar of chocolate, for example, or some lollies, it tastes nice but because it floods our bloodstream with high-GI sugars our body responds by saying we can't tolerate a high blood-sugar level so insulin gets sent in to counteract it. The increased insulin levels cause us to feel hungry again, so we go looking for more food. And what's nearby? Just what we've been munching on!

**Susie:** You are now a motivational speaker. What is your advice?

**Wayne Pearce:** A marathon starts with one step. One step at a time. You've just got to be patient, be patient with whatever you want to achieve in life. Accept responsibility, and just have little goals

STILL HALF MY SIZE

that you set, particularly at the start, just short little goals that you can measure yourself by.

Surround yourself with friends who are supportive, that's real important in every facet of life. If you lie down with dogs, you'll get up with fleas. Enjoy each of your achievements regardless whether they are big or small. You don't have to enjoy it with food, anyone can enjoy it in many ways. If food is the way you celebrate now, find other ways.

**Susie:** And trust yourself?

**Wayne Pearce:** I think people don't realise that they are all natural born achievers. Every single one of us was born to achieve. For example, when we were babies we wanted to crawl, then walk, then run. It didn't matter how many times we fell over when we took our first steps, we kept getting back up again. We just tend to lose that sense of achievement as we get older because we tend to become conditioned to a fear of failure. As we get older we tend to think that if we have a setback, make a mistake or have a failure that we're not worthwhile or we're not good enough.

We need to make mistakes to get better. If you've never failed, all it means to me is that you never step outside your comfort zone, you've never stretched yourself. If we stop making mistakes then we're not doing as much with our lives as we can. Our job is to learn from them.

For more inspiration from Wayne Pearce go to waynepearce.com.au.

# Dave Gorr and Phebe Irwin interview

Dave Gorr and Phebe Irwin were an extremely successful breakfast radio duo on Wave FM Wollongong and got up before the birds to entertain their listeners each weekday for many years, after teaming up in April 2001.

Phebe and Dave proved to be a winning combination. In 2002 after only being together for a year, they won the Commercial Radio Australia 'Best On-Air Team' award, known as a Raward, which is the radio equivalent to our TV Logie awards.

Dave's no stranger to shiftwork since starting his radio career in the 1980s hosting mid-dawn and breakfast shifts on 8DN Katherine in the Northern Territory. He went on to host more mid-dawn and breakfast shifts across Australia including Geelong, Perth, Newcastle, Wollongong and Sydney.

Compared to Dave, co-host Phebe Irwin was a relative newcomer to the early starts associated with shiftwork in breakfast radio, but she had experienced lots of shiftwork while working in the catering industry for a decade before switching careers. Phebe had her first 'taste' of radio at Falls Creek in Victoria and got her start in Albury. In 1997 Phebe started at i98 FM in Wollongong and then joined forces with Dave on Wave FM four years later.

I first met this enormously talented duo at a Bandage Bear benefit night in Wollongong in 2001. Not only were Phebe and Dave both full of life and fun that night, but they were much fuller in size. Both became shadows of their former selves and I welcomed the chance to chat with them to understand their journey and to get some insights into the trials and tribulations that permanent shiftwork had on their health and fitness.

**Susie:** Firstly, what are some of the downfalls to hosting breakfast radio?

**Dave Gorr:** If you want a social life, don't do this job. You can't have a meaningful social life because everyone you want to play with doesn't work the same hours as you. You're sort of thinking about going to bed when everyone else is thinking about going out. Five days a week it starts at 3.30 am then the weekends really muck you up.

**Phebe Irwin:** I'm too tired on Friday nights to do anything, Saturday I'm into the 'normal person routine' again. I stay up past midnight. I reckon I pay though. Sunday night my body is way into the routine and I have to force myself to go to sleep and often can't.

**Dave Gorr:** I think working out in the morning would be the best thing to do because it would start your metabolism for the day and off you go.

**Phebe Irwin:** I also find that if I don't get to the gym as soon as I leave work then I just don't get there. Dave's much more disciplined.

**Susie:** What do you have for breakfast on days when you're working?

**Phebe Irwin:** I try to start with water but I have to have my carbohydrates in the morning.

**Dave Gorr:** Me too. I have to have carbs in the morning as well or I can't deal with it.

**Phebe Irwin:** We have found that it's too hard to do the show without carbs beforehand. You get really vague and you forget what you're doing.

**Susie:** What happens when you come off-air at 9 am?

**Dave Gorr:** Well this morning was typical. At 9 o'clock I had a lovely bowl of cereal, then took a 30-minute break and walked to the shopping centre opposite the station and bought some fruit: bananas and apples usually. I eat these at work before I leave in the afternoon.

**Susie:** And lunch?

**Phebe Irwin:** Lunch can be a movable feast. I used to have something on my way home from the gym, about 1:30 pm, which is usually a sandwich, but they closed the shop (next to the gym). Most days I try and just eat fruit, or maybe some soup or a salad to tide me over but sometimes I'll have a carb attack.

**Dave Gorr:** I usually have something like a sandwich or a bagel. I eat lunch by 2 pm because I go to the gym at 4 pm.

**Susie:** And dinner?

**Phebe Irwin:** Oh, did I mention that I'm lazy! I cooked for so long that these days I am shocking. I'll cook one big thing and make it last, portion it. Like I'll do ratatouille and rice, portion and freeze it and eat that for six weeks. Also, I live right around the corner from a restaurant strip. For about $7.50 I can get stir-fry vegies and rice and I can make that last for two nights. For that price you're not going to get me chopping veggies and cutting and stuff like that.

**Dave Gorr:** I've got a partner so we're generally sitting down for dinner by about 6.30 pm. Tonight it's going to be a lamb curry and last night we had Chinese takeout but usually it's something healthy – steak and salad or some fish and salad. It's usually a salad of some description except tonight when the veggies are in the curry. I've picked up some tricks and tips about cooking from our radio show guests that help to keep my weight down, and our curries are light curries.

**Susie:** So what time's bed?

**Phebe Irwin:** For me, about 8 pm, it depends.

**Dave Gorr:** I go to bed about 8.30 pm to 9 pm.

**Susie:** Do you find shiftwork plays havoc with your body clock?

**Phebe Irwin:** Because your whole life gets turned around you lose the routine and for me if I don't have the routine then the need for convenience takes over and it becomes easy to cheat. Sometimes taking the time necessary to have a good meal can be an inconvenience because you're in the middle of doing something or you're running late for someone or to be somewhere else. So if you're on your way to somewhere it's easy to do drive-through takeaway.

**Dave Gorr:** It's the routine thing for me too. On the weekend I sleep in about three or four hours so I get up around 7.30 am and try to live a normal life, I try and stay up late Friday and Saturday nights.

**Susie:** Do you find your work plays a role in dictating your diet?

**Phebe Irwin:** Yes, for sure. It's a challenge having lunches with clients and listeners. A lot of the time as much as I try to do the right thing we don't choose the menus, and having just started Weight Watchers sometimes I feel quite pressured.

**Susie:** Would you both consider that you had a weight problem?

**Phebe Irwin:** Yes. Definitely. There used to be a joke in the Irwin family, it's the Irwin genes/jeans – one size fits all. Most of my family members are large, and as kids the larger we were the healthier we were within our family – well so the myth goes.

**Dave Gorr:** I don't think I have a weight problem I have a weight challenge and I use my clothes size and how comfortable they are to tell me how I am doing in my challenge. I don't enjoy my clothes being tight and uncomfortable, so they tell me how I am doing.

**Phebe Irwin:** I think one of most challenging things for me about my weight is that I have to get it through my head that I have to exercise at this level for the rest of my life and never go back to eating the way I did in the past. I've also got this stupid fantasy that once I've lost the weight I'll be able to eat nice things again.

I think the big thing for me is to not let the weight 'creep' back on, for me this is always going to be a challenge. I've really got to keep focused on the fact that it's not a matter of being on or off a diet, but that the decision to take control of my weight means a sustained change of lifestyle against years of conditioning.

**Susie:** You both love food, when did that start for you both … as a child?

**Dave Gorr:** I came from a Jewish background so when we were kids there was everything. There was chopped liver, there was wurst, the big fried sausage, great stuff.

**Phebe Irwin:** The Phebe weight story started on the farm with a love of dairy products from a very early age. When we got home from school, Mum would make us egg flips and milkshakes. We moved around a lot until my parents had a sea change and took over the management of a ski lodge, including a chef and bar, at Falls Creek. Living in a ski resort is difficult for kids, I think –

everyone else is on holidays and you just eat and drink like you are too. I think a lot of my bad habits started there.

Eventually I worked as a chef so it was just years and years of preparing food and being a chef that reinforced behaviours learnt earlier.

**Susie:** Did you exercise much in your childhood and teenage years?

**Dave Gorr:** Yeah, I was an oarsman, you know, rowing. I started weight training when I was about thirteen and each year I just got bigger and bigger. I was always Big Dave. After school I continued rowing for years but at age 27 or so, without the intense exercise I started to put on a lot of weight.

**Phebe Irwin:** I can't say I was the svelte athlete. I did ski a bit when we lived at Falls Creek, which was great and exhausting but otherwise not a lot. Nowadays it's a little different but it's hard work as well.

**Susie:** What was your peak weight?

**Dave Gorr:** The heaviest I ever got was about 119–120 kilograms and I'm back down to about 103–104 now. I'd like to be about 95. If I could get down to and stay at 95 kilograms I'd be happy. That's my aim. For my height, 178 centimetres, I should be 87 kilograms but I've got big shoulders, huge legs and it's all from pushing too many weights for too many years.

**Phebe Irwin:** I peaked at well over 120 kilograms. That's when I had my stomach stapled. I had a dramatic weight loss after that, down to around 75 kilograms and kept that off, until I went to the USA and Europe travelling and discovered that through beer, bread and cheese you can stick it back on pretty easily.

**Susie:** Your stomach stapling Phebe, that's a pretty serious step?

**Phebe Irwin:** It is for sure. It was for me, and I'm sure it is for everyone who has the operation. When you first come out of theatre you can only have liquids for days. And this is what they don't tell you, you can liquefy a lot of things that are bad for you or you can live off milkshakes. It doesn't cause miracles to happen, having surgery, it's still up to you.

I have tried many systems, diets and medications since trying to control my weight. I'm an 'expect results now' person and if there's a pill I can take that helps me, then I will, and I think this is one of my failings. Now I accept that only I am responsible for my weight.

I'm now a size 14. That's tremendous as far as I am concerned. I was a size 14 at age fourteen, and only again immediately after my stomach stapling. God, how I remember dreadfully those days at school where I used to wear overalls to school because they were the only clothing that would fit. I am determined not to repeat that, nor anything like it. I enjoy it so much that I can now buy clothes straight off the rack.

**Susie:** Dave, what's the key to controlling your weight?

**Dave Gorr:** Keep it simple I suppose. You've got to exercise so that you balance the amount you take in with the amount of energy you expend. Exercise and some balance in what you eat. Oh, and the routine. Try and find a routine that works for you and, as much as is possible, stick to it.

Sadly Phebe Irwin passed away in August 2014 from complications after an operation. I miss Phebs dearly and will treasure the memories of our catch-ups and lengthy interstate phone calls. Phebe was so funny and smart and the only consolation is knowing she's finally at peace.

# Sandra Sully interview

Sandra Sully is a journalist and one of Australia's favourite newsreaders. Sandra's anchored Network Ten's *Late News* nationally, their *Eyewitness News* bulletin in New South Wales, along with hosting many other TV shows and documentaries.

One of Sandra's little-known talents is that she's a qualified fitness instructor. A small group of us from Channel 10 used to meet up and do a pump class in Bondi Junction some years ago. I felt very spoilt having an instructor out the front and Sandra close by, who would kindly correct me to ensure that I wouldn't injure myself. I learnt more from Sandra, who was also participating in the class, than from the paid instructors in most aerobic classes I've attended.

You've already heard from Phebe Irwin and Dave Gorr about how much an early start impacted on their routine. Sandra talks about her shiftwork experience at the opposite end of the day. Being live on camera she has to look and feel her best and have enough fuel to go the distance.

**Susie:** Please tell me the Sandra Sully story.

**Sandra Sully:** I was born in Brisbane, Queensland and by the time I got through high school I was still pretty unsure of what I wanted to do, so I got a job in the public service while I worked things out. I then worked part-time in a health and fitness business while I studied the industry. I knew I loved it but soon realised it was more of a hobby than a career and so pursued a job in television production, which was the turning point. By then I was studying a Bachelor of Business part-time, but had fallen in love with journalism and switched degrees, and the rest, as they say, is history.

**Susie:** When you spoke about getting into fitness, did you become a qualified instructor?

**Sandra Sully:** Yes, I did. My love of sport and physical education began at an early age. I wanted to try everything and basically did, so by the time I left high school I knew I wanted to work in the industry somehow, but wasn't sure in what capacity. I had some designs on a career, as a Phys. Education teacher but wasn't really ready to study again so I took some time off and began working in the public service.

I started some tertiary study in community recreation and health and also began some part-time work as a gym instructor. I loved the job so much and had all the relevant accreditations so I quickly tossed in the public service and began full-time. It was a really exciting time in the industry as health and fitness was certainly the buzz! I couldn't have been happier being paid to do something I absolutely loved. Gyms were popping up everywhere. I soon moved into management overseeing 5 centres, 25 instructors and 125 exercise classes a week.

**Susie:** Were you always slim and drop dead gorgeous?

**Sandra Sully:** Hardly Susie, but weight was never a major issue for me as I was always so active. I went overseas for a couple of years as an exchange student and on a working holiday and returned a couple of stone heavier. Others were quite surprised. But I just hopped straight back into the gym and got back into shape. I have always felt that health and fitness were a lifestyle choice for me and while that would wax and wane given life's pressures, it would never be a major problem.

**Susie:** As a child, were you a fussy eater?

**Sandra Sully:** No, no, never.

**Susie:** Good on the tooth?

**Sandra Sully:** Susie, I was very good on the tooth. At high school I had a T-bone steak for breakfast and dinner most weekdays. Sure, I was conscious of keeping my weight within certain limits but I was working out so much that it wasn't a major problem. Most days I was either at hockey or gym training before and after school, as well as working as a volunteer gym coach at the local police club. I had a voracious appetite. Banana sandwiches were a favourite plus loads of fruit and of course plenty of chocolate – lots of everything.

**Susie:** How did you know to eat so well?

**Sandra Sully:** Again it stems from your upbringing and I was very fortunate. My family was a very traditional meat and three veg type, but we also loved fresh fruit. I remember traipsing to the markets every week to buy cases of apples, mandarins, grapes and anything else we could get our hands on. My parents couldn't believe how much fruit we ate but were conscious of how important it was to eat well.

Sure, we had loads of 'cheeky' snacks, particularly from my grandmother, but we were all so highly energetic. With two brothers who played a lot of football and spending nearly every winter of my childhood at either a football field, or a netball court or a hockey field, and then the summers at the beach swimming and surfing, we always ate loads of healthy food. We couldn't do what we wanted to do if we didn't.

**Susie:** You mentioned you've always been into fitness. What do you do now, what is your exercise regime now?

**Sandra Sully:** Given my hours it's impossible to participate in team sports so I mostly work-out on my own. Apart from running and swimming I've recently started a little pilates and yoga, which focuses on all the structural imbalances you develop unconsciously from years of sport and never enough stretching! I've also been paying a bit of tennis and golf, which I really love. Golf is fantastic. There are very few sports that get you outdoors for several hours and provide a lifetime of enjoyment. I can play on my own, and often do but what's really neat about golf is that you can play anywhere in the world and with all age groups.

**Susie:** Your exercise routine seems to be constantly evolving, you're adjusting it with your lifestyle rather than being fixed and rigid and if you can't do that, you don't do anything …

**Sandra Sully:** It's a lifestyle choice for me and always has been. I have never seen it as a short-term goal i.e. lose half a stone to fit into a dress and then give up. You have to expect life's hiccups will always be there – ill health, work and family pressures, relationship dramas – but you have to roll with the punches and allow them to bubble through your life and not let the guilt trip beat you. You can't be paranoid or obsessive about missing a session otherwise it'll overwhelm you and that's not the point. You are meant to enjoy it and not be obsessed by it. And you can only do that if the framework is such that it's a lifestyle choice. So if I can't run today and I haven't run this week, it's okay – I've had a really busy week and I'm really tired at the moment but I know in my heart and head that I'll go next week. There are times when I haven't been able to do any exercise for months; it's not the end of the world, because I know I'll get back there – that's life.

**Susie:** So, what would be your best fitness tip?

**Sandra Sully:** My naturopath once said to me, 'If you don't take care of your body, where will you live?' I thought it was one of the most profound things I had ever heard, in that so many people don't see the obvious. It's all about prevention rather than cure. Being conscious of your own health and fitness is the best preventative measure you can take to fend off life's stresses, strains and ailments that seem to be overwhelming this generation and probably generations to come.

A lot of people hide behind the fact that they do so much for everybody else that it becomes an excuse for not doing anything for themselves and they take on the martyr syndrome. You owe yourself half an hour to an hour, a couple of times a week to take responsibility for your own life. It's not a big commitment in any seven days. Why wake up when you are 50 or 60 and say 'I've never had time'? For most people, and I stress not all, that's a cop-out.

**Susie:** What would you eat for breakfast, lunch, dinner and snacks?

**Sandra Sully:** The last couple of years, because of my hours, it's been difficult. I've had to tweak my intake and found that more protein during the day is far more beneficial to my energy levels … so I tend to eat small meals regularly throughout the day. For breakfast I have either a banana smoothie or muesli with soya milk. Lunchtime can be lentil soup, or sashimi, or chicken with a salad. I graze all the time. The trick is having good things to graze on.

**Susie:** Do you have pig-out foods?

**Sandra Sully:** I thought I always had a sweet tooth, but I'm developing a savoury tooth as well, unfortunately! I love ice-cream, peanut M&Ms, chocolate, dips, bread (laughs) … I often pig out, but because I work-out, I can eat most things.

**Susie:** You've been a late-night shiftworker, reading news when most of us were getting ready or already tucked up in bed. How do you keep your energy up at that time?

**Sandra Sully:** I don't eat late. I try to consume most of my meals during a regular day and am very aware of the circadian rhythms that dominate our body's cycle. I try to eat a larger meal late afternoon and then I'll have an early dinner.

**Susie:** Alcohol part of the regime?

**Sandra Sully:** Yeah, I enjoy a drink, absolutely. But everything in moderation. You just have to have a good approach and exercise a bit of discipline. People often think they want a treat, but they want it every day. I think it's important to savour the treat and savour the moment. The treat isn't going to run out, it will be there tomorrow. You might even enjoy it more tomorrow if you wait. (laughs)

**Susie:** Do you have strong willpower?

**Sandra Sully:** I would probably say no, because I have often let myself down, but I think compared to the average bear I probably have more than most.

**Susie:** Can you give us some tips on how to overcome mental obstacles that stop us from achieving our aims and our goals?

**Sandra Sully:** Most people, I think, are fairly selfless. I think you owe it to yourself to be a little selfish, and by that I mean, be kind to yourself. Take a minute or two out of each day for yourself, not just for your own mental health but also for your physical health. Then, when people really need you, you will be better able to give. After a while the martyrdom complex becomes a self-fulfilling prophecy where you live your life for other people and end up being a spent force with nothing left to give. You can give a lot more if it comes from a healthy, strong position. Being positive is the best thing you can bring to any relationship, family or workplace table. I know that's difficult but each and every day it must be the goal. It's easy to drown in a swirl of negativity, but it only pulls you down and everyone else around you.

**Susie:** Any tips on maintaining a healthy lifestyle while shiftworking?

**Sandra Sully:** Unless you are a shiftworker you never fully appreciate how difficult it is and how much it affects your daily rhythms. In some respects I was lucky in that I was brought up in a shiftworking family and know what to expect, but I also now see why my dad was so tired so often. Basically you spend a third of your life in bed so if you deny yourself that time to regenerate you simply won't be able operate at maximum levels. The trick is not to become sleep obsessed but sleep smart … in that you need to recognise you have interrupted the body's natural biorhythms and will need to be clever with your sleeping patterns.

**Susie:** Do you think it important to surround yourself with people who are positive?

**Sandra Sully:** It's really important. Try to discard the negative people in your life, as much as you can and focus on the positive, I can't stress it enough. I don't have any family in Sydney and my friends have been my salvation during my lowest ebbs. I would hate to think where I would be without them.

# Jeff Fenech interview

Nothing has toned my body or changed my shape more than boxing and I was lucky enough to be coached by the best – Jeff Fenech. The three-time world champion at bantamweight, super bantamweight and featherweight is one of the greatest boxers Australia has ever produced. Inducted into the International Boxing Hall of Fame in Canastota, New York, in June 2002, Jeff Fenech is recognised around the world as one of the sporting greats. A controversial draw with African great Azumah Nelson when the majority of the world saw him win, cost Fenech what would have been an amazing fourth world title at super featherweight.

Trained by Johnny Lewis, Fenech was known as the 'Marrickville Mauler' and was like a pocket dynamo in the ring, capturing the hearts of Australian sporting fans with his unique expression, 'I love youse all'.

While Jeff may have hung up his own gloves and retired from professional boxing, it hasn't stopped him from mentoring and creating many more world boxing champions among his Team Fenech boxers.

Who wouldn't jump at the chance to be trained by a three times world boxing champion? Not me, that's for sure. Jeff Fenech shares his story and some fantastic fitness and motivational tips for you.

**Susie:** Please tell us the Jeff Fenech boxing story.

**Jeff Fenech:** I started when I was about seventeen. I never wanted to be a fighter, always wanted to be a footy player and just by coincidence I went to youth club and was pretty fortunate to meet my mate, Johnny Lewis.

Turned professional, October '84, a couple of months after the Olympics and was World Champion in April '85. The shortest time ever, still to this day, for a person to turn from amateur to professional to win a world title, and just everything you see now, just grew from there on. I was learning all the time, like I said. One of the biggest pluses for me was that I was learning all the time because I was still relatively new to the sport and I was getting better every fight, every training preparation.

Won two more titles, had a draw for my fourth, retired, made a comeback, retired and made another comeback and maybe those two comebacks weren't successful but they certainly shaped my life after boxing. I think I learnt more through the comebacks and defeat than I ever did through success. It mightn't have been the most positive thing in my boxing career, but in my life in general, it's the best thing that happened.

**Susie:** Being Maltese, what sort of foods did you grow up on?

**Jeff Fenech:** Rabbit stew, ravioli, pasta – wog food. That's what I still eat today. I was pretty lucky we had a dedicated mum who worked three jobs in the middle of the night and in the day when we were at school, was always there, breakfast, lunch and dinner was always at home, the European way.

**Susie:** Big meals, were you encouraged to have big meals? Were you a big eater?

**Jeff Fenech:** Whatever we wanted, Mum always made more, so if you wanted more and were hungry, we would eat.

**Susie:** Where you always good at sport?

**Jeff Fenech:** Yeah, I was competitive. I don't know whether I was outstanding. Obviously I played footy all my life, I played basketball. I was too small for football, I made all the sides, 'cause I tried hard.

**Susie:** Was it because you were small, do you think, that you developed such drive?

**Jeff Fenech:** No doubt, I always had a chip on my shoulder. I always had to prove I could do what everyone else could do. In life in general, everything you do is all about respect, if you're not respected you can't walk around with your head up high.

**Susie:** Were there ever any times, mentally, that you felt that you just wanted to give up?

**Jeff Fenech:** No, not really. I always enjoyed the adversity, I enjoyed the injuries and stuff. It made people respect me more.

**Susie:** What sort of regime did you follow to stay in shape for boxing?

**Jeff Fenech:** Training every day, twice a day, morning and evening.

**Susie:** I know you watched your intake of bread and potatoes … what about pasta?

**Jeff Fenech:** I ate pasta, but they watched my eating, it was hard. Training was always enjoyable because training for me was like a fight; there was a challenge in that I'd try to better myself every day.

**Susie:** So what do you think makes you fat?

**Jeff Fenech:** Obviously what you eat and drink and the times you consume it. Age makes it harder. As you get older your metabolism changes and that makes it more difficult to lose weight.

**Susie:** We were talking about weight being such an issue in boxing. In fact, as I understand it you went through five weight divisions in boxing …

**Jeff Fenech:** Yeah five divisions but you have to realise they are only four or five pounds to each division, it's not a huge thing. As I said, I grew late. At eighteen or nineteen I was at the Olympics fighting at 51 kilos. At 21, when I won the World Title I was 53 kilos. When I won the World Title in '87 I was 55 ½ kilos, then 57 kilos, 59 and so on.

**Susie:** What key tips do you give to your boxers? You've trained a lot of them in Team Fenech, including Danny Green, what tips do you give them to be a champion?

**Jeff Fenech:** My biggest tip for anybody in any field, whether it's sport or work, is preparation.

**Susie:** I've noticed since training with you that boxing is probably one of the best ways of getting fit and changing your shape and toning, so in that respect it is good for women.

**Jeff Fenech:** Oh, 100 per cent. It's the best thing. If you are doing it with people you know, it is about enjoyment. If you don't enjoy what you are doing then you don't do it. I think what you just said is testimony to what we do up there. We enjoy our training.

**Susie:** I think the reason I came back, aside from the fact that you don't get many offers to be trained by a three-time world boxing champion, was that you didn't fatigue me. The first round I think you let me go 30 seconds and gave me a minute break …

**Jeff Fenech:** That's what I said, there's an art. We're all different. It's about waiting for your client to want to do more, then you can slowly build it up. Had I killed you for the first two weeks, you wouldn't have been back. There's not a chance in the world. You would have showed me that you could do it and then all of a sudden one day just disappeared.

**Susie:** Should you vary your routine in exercise?

**Jeff Fenech:** Of course, variety is the spice of life. It's good to try a few different things here and there. We get used to the same old routine and enjoy it, but it's good to do other things. Like this morning, for instance, we had a day off in the gym and we played touch footy.

# Shelley Taylor-Smith interview

When I think of willpower I'm often reminded of the Gary Puckett and the Union Gap song, 'Lady Willpower' and it could have been easily written for Shelley Taylor-Smith, who has, without a doubt, one of the strongest willpowers I know.

Shelley Taylor-Smith has proven that a champion mindset can make a difference in your life and business. Seven times world champion marathon swimmer, Shelley's male competitors affectionately nicknamed her Dangerous When Wet, which became the title of her best-selling biography.

Setting no less than fifteen world race records, swimming the English Channel and winning the Manhattan Island title in New York City, not once, but five times outright, Shelley Taylor-Smith understands the power of the mind when setting and achieving goals.

**Susie:** Can you tell me the Shelley Taylor-Smith story?

**Shelley Taylor-Smith:** Well, basically I'm an example of a little girl who had a dream and never let go of it. I never had big aspirations and started swimming only because my sister was an asthmatic. My sister is a natural sportsman and I was just a slugger; where she glided I had to battle, but I just had a go. I put in 100 per cent no matter what and I loved every minute of it and so I'd go swimming and I can remember I'd get really excited. Shane Gould was my hero at the 1972 Olympics, and I'd go to bed at night with my swimsuit on. In the mornings, before my dad had even finished jiggling his teabag in his tea cup, I'd be sitting in the car ready to go to swimming training and on the way to the pool I'd have my cap and goggles on; it was a really cool look! Dad would tell me amazing police stories on the way. I would get to the pool motivated and just basically bounding around and my coach would see me coming and go, 'Oh no here she comes, oh and she's still smiling.' So, you know, I just had this passion, this drive. It was great.

**Susie:** So, this little girl swims and trains and achieves what?

**Shelley Taylor-Smith:** You know it was kind of interesting, 'cause I didn't really know I had a handicap until I was about twelve years of age. At twelve we discovered that one leg was markedly shorter than the other. I was then diagnosed with scoliosis. For over 2000 days I wore a back brace, that's five years of my life. It didn't stop me though. Whenever I got out of the shower or out of the pool my mother would put her foot in the middle of my back and strap me into my steel harness. It would bleed raw on my clavicle and my hip and pelvis and I just thought well, I've got the straightest back. I couldn't wait to fling this thing off and go swimming so I could just feel free as a bird. I felt like a caged animal in it. By fourteen I was number one in Australia in the 200 metres backstroke.

**Susie:** You are regarded as one of the world's greatest athletes, achieving victories like number-one world ranking in marathon swimming for both men and women. The first, and to date the last time, a woman in any sport in the world has ever achieved a title like that.

**Shelley Taylor-Smith:** In 1991 when I got the world ranking for number one men and women, I won the race in Sydney Harbour. Who knows why we were sharing the same ranking but we were. We did not even have equal prize money back then, and you know, we all started together and all finished together. What's the big deal?

My training partners were always men. In marathon swimming, it's always been that we all start together and we share the prize money, so in 1991 when I came out first I thought 'Oh good, that's really cool, I did it.' I didn't think anything of it. I've never been one to rest on my laurels. I have always believed you are only as good as your last swim so I always focused on the next event. We debriefed, celebrated of course, and then said 'Next!'

Recently I was doing a school talk and one kid asked 'What's it like to be the best in the world?' I did not have an answer and was flabbergasted. I eventually answered that it wasn't about being number one, it was about being number one in my own world and achieving what I wanted. Achieving my dreams.

**Susie:** So were you always good at sport?

**Shelley Taylor-Smith:** I just had a go. I played netball and softball and all those sports growing up at school. I wasn't fantastic but was always into school sports teams, whether it was weekend netball or whatever. I just loved team sports because swimming wasn't really a team sport in those days.

**Susie:** How much of it is mental?

**Shelley Taylor-Smith:** Come race day, for me, probably 100 per cent. I can remember my first world record was in 1983, we were swimming in the lake as pre-season training at the University of Arkansas and I beat all the men. A week later I broke the world record by about 40 minutes and I was part of the women's relay and the men's relay. I went to the boot of my car and grabbed an esky with champagne and glasses.

My coach asked where I got it from, and I replied that 'I had a dream last night I would do it and you always taught me that if I fail to prepare, I prepare to fail, so I looked at my checklist and I didn't have 'celebrating' covered so I went and got the champagne, 'cause I just knew I was going to do it!'

**Susie:** You've had some down times though; in 1980 you nearly died when you were crushed from the rear by a truck, leaving you with whiplash and permanent lower-back damage. Were there any times where you just wanted to give up?

**Shelley Taylor-Smith:** Yeah, when you talk about my turning points or the lowest lows, which in hindsight became my highest highs, my dad's death was a huge blow to me at fifteen years of age

Later, I was 23 and in Arkansas, in traction and being turned like a chicken on a spit, and I didn't get [how serious it was] until one day when they lowered my medication and my doctor said, 'We've got a major problem. You've severed the nerves of the spine at L5 and S1. We cannot find any neurological activity from the waist down, you don't know that we are scraping your feet every day and there is no reaction.'

Tears were pouring down my face and my dad's voice came to me, 'Get back up, have a go, doesn't matter if you fall over. Get back up, brush yourself off, have another go.' It was probably what I thought was my gold medal moment in life. I remember getting up, taking my first step walking, it was not a great step but it was a step, and realising this I got so excited I peed my pants! I did get back up and I got walking, I shuffled for twelve months to class.

**Susie:** Do you have to watch your weight?

**Shelley Taylor-Smith:** I've probably looked at my body more times than most people in their lives because every day I put a swimsuit on, morning and night. So I was so aware whether things were tucked in and straps were right, were my nipples even. I didn't even have to weigh myself in being conscious about my weight.

**Susie:** You've taken on a whole new fitness regime … and not so much weight loss, but certainly centimetre loss.

**Shelley Taylor-Smith:** Yeah. When I work with people, I try to have them focus on what they want to be instead of having them think about what they want to lose, so I applied this to myself. Because my schedule is so chaotic, I didn't have a routine, and as a consequence a few things got out of whack and I became uncomfortable with how I felt about me. So I set a goal for this year, to be happy with how I felt.

Now, I like the way my clothes fit, I like the way I look in a swimsuit. It was not so much about how everybody else felt; it was about how I felt about me. I feel really good in my skin.

I am disciplined, once I find something. It was about getting back to basics and getting back into my skin again. So I just sat down with someone and said 'This is what I'm doing' and they said 'This is what you need to do.' It was about what I needed to focus on.

I've never actually been on diets except for carbohydrate loading for swimming and protein building. I now have a carbohydrate and protein drink with omega-three oils in the morning with fresh fruit. The rest of the day is green tea and lots of nuts for protein for morning and afternoon tea. Lunch

is chicken or tuna and as much deep green salad as I want –
whether it's bok choy or whatever – then steak, fish or chicken at
night. I drink two to three litres of water per day and heaps of
green tea and if I get the munchies, I have another protein shake.
Really basic and easy.

**Susie:** You have incredible willpower. Can you train yourself, or does
it come naturally?

**Shelley Taylor-Smith:** I know a lot of people who have gone
bankrupt and have gone on to be very, very successful people
and a lot of people with disabilities and everything and it comes
down to our minds. Mind over matter. Remember, our mind
doesn't know the difference between creative imagination and
real fact. So if you tell yourself you are good at something, if
you tell yourself enough times, you'll believe it. And that's the
unfortunate thing in relationships or if you've been brought up
saying you're fat, you're ugly, too short etcetera and what happens
is if you listen to it long enough you believe it. Whether it's a fact
or not you believe it and you will act on it. The greatest gift you
can give yourself is allowing yourself to create whatever you want
in your life and that comes from the power of the mind.

**Susie:** Can you give us some tips on how to overcome some mental
obstacles that might be keeping people from their goals and aims
and objectives?

**Shelley Taylor-Smith:** Probably the first thing is to treat any obstacle
as a positive, not a negative. If you don't have any problems, then
that's a problem. A problem, an obstacle, is something that you
have to create energy in order to move around. If people are
feeling stagnant, it's because they don't have enough obstacles or
aren't challenging themselves.

Embrace your obstacles and say what can I learn from you,
which will allow me to let go of the problem I've got right now,
and then stuff it and crush it. Once crushed, turn to the future,
leaving the obstacle behind in both fact and emotion.

**Susie:** Is there a champion in everyone?

**Shelley Taylor-Smith:** Absolutely. Absolutely. Because the core of
who we are is absolute joy and completeness and wholeness. It is

our birthright to be the champion of our own world! There's no fear, no anger, no sadness, no guilt, there's no comparison to anyone else.

**Susie:** Any tips for creating your champion mindset?

**Shelley Taylor-Smith:** Yeah, be positive. All the power to be positive is available to you now. The power comes from within and it's about realising that you can cope whenever you want when you know the power comes from within. It's nice to know that you can do it with your own power. Also the power of NOW. Being 100 per cent present in everything that you do. So many of us go back to our past and drag that baggage with us into our future.

For details of Shelley Taylor-Smith's Champion Mindset books, seminars and Taylor-made solutions go to championmindset.com.au.

# John Maclean interview

One person who has shown me better than most how you can overcome huge obstacles and come back even stronger mentally, physically, emotionally and spiritually is the extraordinary athlete John Maclean.

John's dream, being a natural sportsman all his life, was to play first-grade rugby league for the Penrith Panthers. In 1988, when he'd only recently turned 22, John was bike training for a triathlon when he was hit by an eight-tonne truck travelling at 120 kilometres an hour. In the accident, John broke his back in three places, pelvis in four, right arm in two, suffered a fractured sternum, broken ribs, punctured lung, closed head injury and ripped the right knee off the bone. John lost so much blood he shouldn't have lived. But live he did.

John was born in Cronulla, the youngest of three children, who only ever wanted to be as good as his older brother at sport and follow in his footsteps.

In his wheelchair, Paralympian John Maclean exceeded even his own sporting expectations and what he's achieved since, which I'll reveal at the end of this interview is nothing short of astonishing!

**Susie:** What were you like at school? Were you always good at sport?

**John Maclean:** I was naturally gifted at sport; I won everything I did in sport although I didn't apply myself outside of sport at school – which I am working on now. Then after leaving school my goal was to play first-grade football and to get a job as a fireman and enjoy work and sport.

**Susie:** Your accident was devastating physically. What saved you?

**John Maclean:** Looking back, when the ambulance took me to the hospital the surgeon said to my father that I wasn't expected to live. Acknowledging I had great medical care, I survived from a burning desire from within, saying to myself that I don't want to die, so that's what got me through. I was a couple of days in a coma, a couple of weeks in intensive care and four months all up in North Shore Hospital.

Some amazing things happened. The first was my decision not to die. They told me I had more broken bones than all the other people in the spinal unit put together. Later, I was moved from intensive care to the general ward. Being wheeled into the general ward I thought I was pretty pathetic and then I realised the other three guys in the room were all quadriplegics, high-level quadriplegics, meaning assistance for everything.

This was a 'light-bulb moment' for me – never to feel sorry for myself. I am lucky for two reasons: I lived and I am not a quadriplegic.

The third thing that happened was a little reverse psychology our family doctor used on me when he visited shortly after I was moved into the general ward. He looked at me and said, 'Don't worry, you're going to be bigger, stronger and faster than you were before the accident' and then left. He planted a very strong and deep seed. I made a decision right there and then to push myself as hard as possible so that my nerves would have the best chance at regenerating.

My accident and hospitalisation have been a constant motivation, an inspiration to keep on going. So when things are tough for me I think back to those guys who would love to have the opportunity to go through that discomfort in a different way.

**Susie:** How about mentally? Were there ever times when you felt like giving up?

**John Maclean:** Never.

**Susie:** Even through all the pain?

**John Maclean:** The discomfort that I went through in hospital and later was unbearable but going through such a high level of pain, you can start to appreciate still having the joy to feel pain. At times the pain revisits me, even today.

Life for me took a right-hand turn when I got hit by that truck and it's shown me a whole new direction. It's taken me many years to actually say to you that this is a gift. I didn't see the clarity in that for many years and finally I've taken the opportunity to slow down and have a look at myself.

I feel that I needed to go through all those experiences prior to my accident to have the fortitude and the strength of character and will to be able to make that transition and play the best that I can with the cards I've been dealt.

**Susie:** Does willpower play a part and if so where do you find it?

**John Maclean:** Yes. The willpower comes from an internal drive to succeed in whatever I set my mind to.

**Susie:** How important is it to find yourself?

**John Maclean:** I think that's the essence of life. To me that's what it's all about. Accept the cards you're dealt but they're not an excuse either. Try and use the things that do go wrong as ways of learning more about the person who lives inside of you.

**Susie:** So your accident was a beginning not an end?

**John Maclean:** Absolutely! After sustaining my injuries I found myself at a juncture and had to choose a new path. I think I have had a richer and far more rewarding life than the one I had planned as a rugby-league player and fireman. Looking back now, I completed the Hawaiian Ironman, the English Channel, Olympic and Paralympic Games, Sydney to Hobart Yacht Race and have raised nearly a million dollars for kids in wheelchairs by hand cycling from Brisbane to Melbourne.

**Susie:** The third time you completed in the Hawaiian Ironman you did it within the 'able bodied' cut-off time. Was that important to you?

**John Maclean:** The objective was from the start that if I could go to Hawaii, which is the toughest endurance event in the world, and make all the cut-off times in a wheelchair then I could go down any street in the world and I would feel complete. But within myself I had to keep on going until I'd made all the cut-off times just for myself.

**Susie:** You bulked up big time for the English Channel swim and when you finished you lost 20 kilograms in six weeks to get ready for the Paralympics. How did you do it?

**John Maclean:** My dietitian told me that if I didn't put on weight then there was no way I'd make the Channel because the water's so cold – fourteen to fifteen degrees. Apparently a lot of swimmers who aren't carrying enough fat suffer hypothermia and have to pull out. I realised that I seriously had to put some weight on so I ate lots and lots and lots of food and I managed to put on 20 kilos over a period of probably four to five months.

I swam 15 kilometres a day training for the English Channel swim. Ten kilometres in the morning and three to five at night.

**Susie:** You gained this weight, swam the English Channel but then you couldn't rest on your laurels and take it off over five months, you had to lose it all in five weeks.

**John Maclean:** After the Channel I already knew that I wanted to be part of the Paralympics in Sydney and represent my country in wheelchair racing, that's the most competitive sport. When I got back I fasted for a week so that was water for the first two days, then the next two to four days was water plus fruit and then five and six was water and fruit and vegetables. I've got to tell you I've never felt that good in my life because I had all this energy stored in my body. I didn't need to put any more energy in; the car was full of petrol, if you're using that analogy. Or maybe it was a truck for me at the time (laugh). I felt fantastic. I didn't need to sleep much.

**Susie:** Didn't you find you were falling over if you only had water for the first two days?

**John Maclean:** No, I mean I was certainly hungry but given that all the carbohydrates that were stored in the pancreas, that's the energy that one needs. [After my week of fasting] I was putting the protein in to keep me going but I had the fuel there. I realised the first thing I needed to do was to lose a whole lot of weight before I could get into my racing chair. Then I needed to learn how to push it properly, then I needed to go fast and obviously I needed to get a coach and I needed to go fast enough to get qualifying, so I had some work ahead of me to do.

I then just had some proteins. I went back to the dietitian. I can't speak for others, but for me, because I had so much excess weight on, I had basically chicken, fish and steak, fruit and vegetables, simple carbs. Eating the right types of food and exercise I was then able to drop the weight.

It's input versus output. At the start when I needed to put the weight on I was putting more calories in than I was burning. So when I wanted to lose it, it was not putting the calories in and increasing the output, which was exercise and it fell off again. But I've been very regimented, very strict and I needed to be overweight for the swim but I didn't like the look of it when I'd finished with it so it came off quite quickly.

**Susie:** What about the fat? Things like chocolate or milk products or cheese?

**John Maclean:** No because I'd put so much of that into my system, which equalled me getting 20 kilos heavier, I didn't need to put that in again. And prior to that I've always been fairly healthy and been conscious of body image and things like that so I didn't have that as a goal to losing that weight. That was food that was not going to serve me. I viewed myself as being somewhat of a racing machine if I was going to be competitive for sport. You need to put the right fuel in the car to get the best performance so no, none of those foods that you've suggested.

**Susie:** What's your eating regime?

**John Maclean:** It changes, depends on how I'm feeling at the time. For me I am conscious of my body image and what I'm about to do. I am about to do an Ironman again so I know that if I don't put the right food in I won't have the energy to keep on training hours on end.

There are times at the moment, in the morning, when I enjoy having a herbal tea and fruit and I'll have fruit again at lunchtime. So I'm just eating clean types of foods because I'm going through an energy period and I want to make sure that I'm feeling good all the time.

**Susie:** By clean foods, I take that as whole foods as opposed to processed foods? How do they alter your energy levels?

**John Maclean:** If you've ever had chips with salt or too much salt or sugar, what generally happens is you get a spike so it gives you a bit of a lift and you feel the benefit of that. That's very similar to some of these caffeinated drinks, whether they're V's or Red Bull, all this sort of stuff gives you an instant high – the caffeine, guarana and all the rest of that – but on the other end of that it brings you lower than what you were. So clean food to me means that you are eating the sort of foods that will be able to sustain you through the day. That's what I'm looking at right now.

A perfect example while it's quite cool is porridge. Have your porridge in the morning with fruit and herbal tea. Anything that's caffeinated – tea, coffee, guarana and that type of thing – again give you that lift and then bring you lower than what you were. So I'm trying to find stuff that works for me throughout the course of the day.

When I'm feeling like a snack, instead of having a coffee and a muffin, I would have a herbal tea and maybe a handful of nuts or nut mix, which also has raisins and things like that. And if I'm still feeling hungry I'll have a piece of fruit. So those sorts of foods that sustain you throughout the course of the day to keep your energy at the optimum level.

I'm a big believer, to divert just briefly, that if one can manage their energy, they can manage their life. For most people in the corporate world, the afternoon between three and four o'clock, that's their downtime, so there's not a lot of productivity. And that's because they have either had a large lunch, or they've had a high sugar/caffeine content in the body and they're feeling the low effects of that.

If one was to have the energy type foods that keep them on the same course throughout the day they'd feel a lot better for that and have the energy to partake in all aspects of life. So nutrition is very important.

**Susie:** Fast foods are often high in fat, sugar, salt but it's often easier and cheaper to eat badly.

**John Maclean:** Those so-called convenience foods, it's easier to drive in and buy them but I'm aware – and we all have choices – I'm aware of what's in lots of those types of foods and I also know that when I've eaten those types of food I don't feel good. I generally don't feel good so it's telling me that something's not right and it's very rare that I would stop in and eat something that I wouldn't normally eat. Very rare. I'd have to be starving to get close to that.

John Maclean has gone onto achieve what most thought was impossible. In 2016, after 25 years in a wheelchair happily competing and exceeding even his own expectations in every sport he conquered, John undertook a comprehensive NeuroPhysics training and rehabilitation program with founder Ken Ware, which has seen the first worldwide account of a medically defined paraplegic being able to walk again unassisted.

Those who know how incredibly committed and focused John Maclean becomes with any project he undertakes, won't be surprised to learn that John was able to walk again in an unprecedented time scale of just four sessions. I have no doubt John Maclean will keep rewriting the text and history books with all his future achievements as he continues to inspire.

You can read more about John Maclean's motivating story on his website johnmaclean.com.au.

# Tara Moss interview

Tara Moss is a critically acclaimed award-winning author, journalist, TV documentary presenter, speaker, human rights advocate, anti-cyberbullying campaigner and mother. Since 1999 she has written eleven bestselling books, published in nineteen countries and thirteen languages. She is a PhD candidate at the University of Sydney and has earned her private investigator credentials (Cert III) from the Australian Security Academy. Her latest book is *Speaking Out: A 21st Century Handbook for Women and Girls*. Tara is an outspoken advocate for human rights and the rights of women and children. She has been a UNICEF Goodwill Ambassador since 2007.

Tara's one of Australia's top crime writers, successfully making the transition from international top model to an international shooting-star of popular crime fiction.

Tara is not only the epitome of style, grace, charm, and beauty, she's also intelligent, witty and very insightful. Don't worry, she's not perfect. Surprising as it may seem, there are a number of things Tara can't do and one of them is cooking.

When she's not penning her next award-winning thriller or jet setting around the world on a book tour or researching her next tome, she's busy being a wife and mum. I wanted to know how someone with no culinary skills and who lives in the fast lane out of a suitcase and in restaurants could stay so trim, taut and terrific

**Susie:** Please tell me the Tara Moss story.

**Tara Moss:** The Tara Moss story? I hope it's just getting started.

I started writing when I was about ten years old back in British Columbia, Canada. I went on a fabulous tangent modelling after someone told me I should model because I was already six feet tall and only fourteen years of age. I was built like a beanpole at the time, which is hard to imagine now.

Writing is my passion, yet I didn't think of it in a professional context, or as something that I'd be able to turn to after I'd finished modelling. I finally got up the courage to enter a short story in a competition called the Scarlet Stiletto Awards. I was very lucky and won the young writers' award for my short story 'Psycho Magnet'. That was the first professional encouragement I'd had as a writer.

Around that time Selwa Anthony, my agent, contacted me and asked what else I was working on and when I said a novel called Fetish she asked that I send it to her when finished. So I suddenly had to treat the book a little bit more seriously. About six months later I gave her the manuscript that I had completed. She read it over, and loved it. HarperCollins eventually published it. So that changed my life quite significantly. It was a real reinforcement of what I already loved. Naturally, I didn't recognise that I might have a talent for it, I just had a passion for it. But as we all know, passion is an important ingredient, because if you love something so much you get good at it over the years, before anyone has any idea that you're doing it. My passion for writing hasn't lessened at all.

**Susie:** Were you a fussy eater?

**Tara Moss:** Never. I eat everything. In fact I remember lunch times in school I hated most of the food my mum would give me, like sandwiches. Sandwiches are so boring I wanted cookies and I could have eaten cereal with sugar all over it three times a day when I was a kid. I have a sweet tooth but then again I have a savoury tooth as well, I just have big teeth, let's face it!

**Susie:** Do you have to watch your weight?

**Tara Moss:** Now I don't. I eat pretty much everything. I think it was harder when I was a teenager because I was modelling. I still had that silly thing that a lot of kids have, which is that you want to please everyone. I've since grown out of it, but none the less you're a kid, you're impressionable, people are telling you 'Oh you've got to be this size' and that was the first time I'd ever thought about it. I was about sixteen at the time I started to fill out as a woman, and the agency sort of went 'Uh oh, hang on, hang on. We like your look as it is, which is very androgynous.' And they didn't want me to change, which is impossible. I'm just not the body type. Look at my folks and they all looked like me.

I have a Dutch background – tall, big shoulders, big boobs, big teeth, big grin, and lots of hair. We're not little people, we're not waifish. When I started to become that at sixteen, there was some pressure and I tried a couple of those awful fasting diets, which masqueraded as being healthy.

I'm against dieting now. I think it's a terrible thing because it's not a lifestyle, it's a goal. It's short-lived and often dangerous. I think it is also very bad for your self-esteem to imagine you are not okay as you are. If you have health problems change your lifestyle, don't diet.

**Susie:** So what do you think makes you fat?

**Tara Moss:** First of all what's fat? If you are medically fat you are doing the wrong things to yourself. That is lifestyle. If you've got a different body type to someone else you are not necessarily fat, and I think that's a very important distinction, because I see a lot of really beautiful women who humble themselves mentally all the time because they are unhappy with what they've been given. And they're beautiful. They are gorgeous and any man would tell them they're gorgeous but they don't listen, because they don't look like something in a particular magazine they happen to like. I think that's a real tragedy.

**Susie:** What do you cook?

**Tara Moss:** I don't cook at all. I don't cook, and that's actually not an exaggeration People go 'Oh yeah yeah yeah, but what do you cook?' I say no, I actually don't.

**Susie:** What eating plan do you live by?

**Tara Moss:** I don't live by many plans. Certainly not an eating plan. I might have breakfast at home. I might have cereal or something that involves no cooking, then the rest of the day I might eat out. And now I have a wonderful husband who cooks for me, so sometimes I eat at home. I eat probably more meals at home now than I have ever before, but that still means about three nights at home and four nights in restaurants or with friends having dinner. Mark is a fabulous cook and he's totally comfortable with that and so am I, so it works wonders.

Cooking has never been a focus of mine. It wasn't an issue, it wasn't a problem, and so I never changed it. Then when I started writing, I thought every meal preparation was a chapter I could be writing. I don't cook, I don't iron, I don't do certain things because I can work and I can take myself out for a nice meal when I've done a good job. That is the way I prefer things right now. Perhaps when I am less busy that may change.

**Susie:** What would you eat breakfast, lunch and dinner?

**Tara Moss:** Eggs and bacon, cereal, muesli, you name it for breakfast. Lunch could be anything – chicken Caesar salad, steak sandwich, pasta and soup – pretty much anything that exists on menus I'll eat. Apart perhaps from things that are very obviously fast food and dripping with unhealthiness.

I don't go into any fast food restaurants; I don't go into chain restaurants. I think no matter where you live if you walk down to the local restaurant that's owned locally, by people who love food, and you're going to do a whole lot better than you are walking down the street to the local chain restaurant. It's nothing to do with calories; it's just to do with the realness of the nutrients still in the food.

**Susie:** What about snacks and treats?

**Tara Moss:** Yeah bring it on! Chocolate, fruit, muesli bars, smoothies, anything.

**Susie:** Alcohol?

**Tara Moss:** Love alcohol. Alcohol's my friend. I love it, it's great. Moderation though, of course.

**Susie:** What's your pig-out food?

**Tara Moss:** I love chocolate, anything with chocolate in it, especially when it's that time of the month. Sometimes I am driven by the need for chocolate, and that is just fine by me. The other thing is that my husband's figured out that I become an angry bear when I haven't eaten. I eat a lot all day. I need to eat a lot of meals as I go. So between now and lunch I'll probably have something, a smoothie or bar of something or muffin or whatever and then I'll eat lunch. And then I'll have something before dinner and then

I'll have something for dinner and something after dinner. That is just me.

If I ever get to five hours between actually eating things, the first thing I do is go vague, my brain doesn't work as well, I'm not getting enough sugar to my brain. I become vague and then the emergency thing happens – I get really tense and believe me it's not nice. I've got to get food into me and my body is telling me 'Emergency! Eat! Now!'

**Susie:** How does all the travelling you do impact on your routine and your health and fitness?

**Tara Moss:** It throws you off but I've never been one who's had routines so I probably don't feel it as much as other people might. I don't have a background of things being normal or routine driven. I don't have regular habits that I do every day that when they're gone throw me off kilter.

**Susie:** How do you keep fit and how often?

**Tara Moss:** I have acute scoliosis. My back is very crooked. I've actually got the spine of a six-foot-two person jammed into the body of a six-foot person. I've got an inch or two inches of spine going all weird directions in my middle, so that is certainly my weakest physical link, and it has been for a long time. I've seen back specialists every couple of weeks since I was about fourteen.

Eventually we came across the idea that I might be able to strengthen my back with the right sort of exercise. I'd been doing exercise, but perhaps not the right stuff. But now I've got a personal trainer, and he is brilliant for what I need. I might do a session for an hour a week, focused on core stability. It's not a lot to ask. It's helped me enormously and I haven't been crippled since. In fact I haven't seen a back specialist now for about six months, which is a first since I was a little girl. That's because kickboxing, physical boxing, core stability work for me. I also do other stuff if I can. Often I can't. I also love to cycle. I do maybe 50 minutes on the bike four days a week on local bike paths if I can. I also love to kayak here and in Canada. It is a beautiful sport.

**Susie:** And how many books are left in Tara Moss?

**Tara Moss:** At least one every two years until I croak. Time is a problem for me, not ideas.

For more on Tara Moss and her latest books and blogs go to taramoss.com.

# Trevor Hendy interview

I had a plethora of interesting and knowledgeable people cross my path during all the talkback radio shifts I did on Radio 2GB. One of those was former Ironman Trevor Hendy, who co-wrote *Shape Up Australia* with his good friend Olympic swimmer Samantha Riley. Trevor believes that an holistic understanding of your body, mind and soul will help you set your goals and achieve them. Trevor is very much a family man and I also asked him what sort of influence he has over his four children's health and wellbeing.

**Susie:** How did Trevor Hendy get to this point, what are your roots?

**Trevor Hendy:** I was born in Melbourne in 1968 and my parents left Victoria when I was three and travelled around Australia for two years with just my sister, who's five years older, and me. Dad was trying to find a place that he felt was the place to raise the family, and he didn't feel that Melbourne, even though he had everything there, was that place.

We ended up on the Gold Coast. I joined Nippers when I was eight years old and then the rest is kind of a progression from there. I was a really shy kid and having people pointing at you and looking at you and all that sort of stuff is like, no way not for me. I remember I cried my first day, didn't want to go, I hated the thought of competition, but something changed and I ended up enjoying it. I always tell the story that I won the beach flags on my first day because it sounds better but I think I might have come second really. I enjoyed the feeling you get when everyone's so happy with you when you do well.

At about sixteen a world-champion coach came up from South Australia and somewhere in the back of my mind I just thought, 'Right I can do this.' So I started training and a year later I was the Australian champion for board paddling and second runner up in the under-nineteen Ironman. Then a year later I became runner up again and then I won an open title so I was the second youngest person to do that and it all kind of happened in about two and a half years.

**Susie:** Were you always good at sport?

**Trevor Hendy:** No, no, definitely not, probably not until about high school. End of primary school, start of high school I noticed a couple of times I could run well because I'd run in the cross country races or the fifteen hundreds and I'd do really well in those. But no, other than that, I started playing tennis when I was about fourteen and made it into the Ken Rosewall tennis squad and that was just over here, we lived around the corner. I played quite well and ended up playing quite competitive tennis but I couldn't get my head around the competition side. So I could win in the club thing, but if I went over to a regional competition, I'd get beaten six love six one. I just had trouble competing out there in the real world.

**Susie:** How much of it then is mental?

**Trevor Hendy:** Once upon a time I would have said 90 per cent, now I think a little bit differently because I've discovered you have to look at the mental, emotional and spiritual aspects of your life. I have learnt within myself or I feel within myself that we do create our own luck, you know, we do create situations to happen for us. If we're in the right place, as in our own heart, then the things we want unfold. And that's what I felt with Ironman; I was meant to come through and learn so much from that sport because things did unfold; I had some magic days in that sport. I think there's a bit bigger picture to it than just the mental side. I'd go to a race on a day of huge surf and my coach helped me incredibly, looking at things in a way that I didn't.

**Susie:** In your book *Shape Up Australia,* which you co-wrote with Samantha Riley, you talk about taking a holistic approach to getting into shape.

**Trevor Hendy:** It would have been so easy for me to be specific and really go all out and make a training manual because I know that back to front. Training is not the only thing that got me to where I was and that's what I later discovered. I was looking at life in a sort of more holistic sense when I sat down to write that book and the funny thing was the book ended up being very general and very broad and very open – almost like you could read it in twenty years' time.

**Susie:** What do you eat? You're pretty disciplined aren't you?

**Trevor Hendy:** Yeah it's funny with the word discipline. I hunger for what I need so I used to literally eat fourteen Vita Brits. So for breakfast the fourteen Vita Brits have disappeared now – I'm down to about two to three Vita Brits a day with some Sports Plus on top. Occasionally toast, very rarely bacon and eggs and stuff. I always felt like that wasn't a breakfast meal. I don't know why. I know a lot of protein diets that I have tried for a while, it just didn't feel like a breakfast meal to me.

Lunch is usually sandwiches or left over pasta, still much the same as I used to have. I like a balance, bit of fried food you know. A little mini spring roll one or two of those and a dim sim when I'm flying past the shop – it's the oils or something.

Dinner, we eat very well for dinner, we always have. We might have steamed fish, we might have seafood once a week. If I feel like a seafood hit we'll have salmon sashimi and I'll go and hand select it and put the Japanese love into it, and cut it all up. Then we have probably two lots of chicken a week, maybe one lot of lamb a week, and maybe a roast every now and then. Beef, maybe steak, once every second week or something. So every now and then I need a steak and I get the biggest T-bone and have it and then I think, yes, whatever I needed out of that steak I got it. And pastas and things like that so I think somewhere it all fits in, balanced.

**Susie:** What are your treats?

**Trevor Hendy:** I love dark chocolate – it's very much a thing for me. Nestle Club have this amazing range now and they have the peppermint cream one and they have almond, they have fruit and nut and they have this dark and white one.

**Susie:** How often would you treat yourself to that?

**Trevor Hendy:** Jo only looked in the fridge last night and said, 'You're eating a lot of chocolate lately.' A lot of chocolate is probably not much at all, maybe three or four rows of chocolate a day, but lately I think probably every second or third day I've gone through a family block.

**Susie:** What sort of health and fitness advice are you now passing on to your children?

**Trevor Hendy:** I'm working with my kids to get their own answers and their own understanding and not trying to put in my limiting viewpoints. I'm very aware of not locking them into a whole heap of false beliefs which I've sort of opened my eyes to in recent times. So I'm trying to work in both ways with them so we just talk about the energy of your body and how much energy you can get. And we talk to them about food and anger and happiness and all those sort of things. And on the food side we say, look it's good to have snacks and treats but you've got to check with yourself whether that's going to really make your body healthy for the day. We pack them a very healthy lunch and make sure they have a healthy breakfast in the morning. Healthy dinner at night, but we do treat them.

**Susie:** Do we need to put ourselves first a lot of the time?

**Trevor Hendy:** At one level we need to realise we need to put ourselves first but there's that old rule that you can't look after someone else unless you've looked after yourself. You fasten your own mask before you help others in the aeroplane, that sort of thing. So I think, yes we do need to look after ourselves but we need to ask ourselves, is the step I'm taking good for the people around me as well?

**Susie:** You say you never exercise.

**Trevor Hendy:** To me, working with people and even when I was doing competitive sport, that's not exercising; it's just what you do so that you can do what your body needs. Maybe if you are just happy within yourself and do what your body needs, maybe that's exercise.

**Susie:** Have you ever had any self-esteem issues?

**Trevor Hendy:** I think so. There was a time when I was in that classic thing of trying to prove myself as a man as well. There are a lot of messages we get in life. I've got friends that have been super famous in different areas and people say, 'Oh I wish I was like that person.' Yet I know the rich and famous are going through exactly the same things as me, you and everyone else out there. So to me that relates back to self-esteem. And it relates back to whether you truly are happy and comfortable with yourself or not.

**Susie:** To wrap up, what are some of the tips that you can give to overcome those mental obstacles that do prevent us from achieving our goals and our aims?

**Trevor Hendy:** Number one, it's good to decide that me, myself, I'm going to do it. When you make positive decisions and commit to them, and I mean you really commit to them, then the world will back you moving in the right direction. Don't let compromising thoughts from anyone else or from yourself come in and take you off track. If they do creep in be okay with it, look at it, learn from it and take charge of it, and don't let it take charge of you. But head in a direction that's right for you and ultimately you will find people that will head with you; you'll learn the right things from the right people and just stay true to yourself.

Details of Trevor Hendy's Boot Camp for the Soul are at trevorhendy.com.

# Jessica Rowe interview

I adore every chance I get to sit alongside the fabulous Jessica Rowe as a co-host on *Studio 10*, when I frequently fill in for regular hosts Ita Buttrose and Denise Drysdale. We have polarising opinions and don't always agree with each other but Jess's heart is always in the right place. She is one of the nicest, most genuine people I know.

When we were both at Network Ten the first time round, we saw each other very regularly but were like 'ships that pass in the night' as we shared a dressing room in their Sydney studios in the late 1990s–early 2000s. I was working on my dream job on *Good Morning Australia* with Bert Newton and Jess was excited to be in her first news-presenting role and had not long been married to her husband Peter Overton.

Back then it was distressing to watch Jess cop such a barrage of media speculation from time to time that she was anorexic, just for being so tall and slim. I've been in Jessica's company socially and on set and watched her be the first to sample the various dishes cooked up on *Studio 10*. She has a very healthy appetite and wisely just cops the criticism on the chin. But nonetheless we both recognise how damaging these taunts can be on your self-worth no matter what your size and shape.

I took the opportunity to chat with Jess for my first book about being on the other side of the spectrum. I know you'll glean a great deal from her sensible approach to health, fitness and life in general.

**Jessica Rowe:** I've been a news presenter at Channel 10 for eight and a half years now. I love it; it's my dream job. When I was in high school I wanted to be a journalist, I wanted to work on television, I wanted to be a news presenter. To me, television is such a powerful medium and I think, it sounds a bit naive, but I wanted to make some sort of small difference. I thought by being a journalist, by informing people about the world round them, what was going on, that might be some small way to make a difference and contribute.

**Susie:** Did you do any sort of training?

**Jessica Rowe:** I did. When I finished school, I took a year off. I had great fun, I sort of bummed around and worked in coffee shops and clothes shops and had fun and learned a bit more about myself. Then I moved to Bathurst in western New South Wales and went to university there and did a Communications degree.

**Susie:** And you've done study since then?

**Jessica Rowe:** Yes, I've done a Masters of International Studies at Sydney Uni, which I found so inspiring and interesting. With my work I go through the same routine each day, of course the news is different every day, but I was looking for more intellectual challenges. So I thought, often we would report on things that almost seemed to be in isolation, world events, Middle East. But there is always so much history that has gone up to that event happening and I thought I wanted to learn more about the world around me, and especially the world I'm talking about, reporting on. So I did the Masters part-time and I think it took about four years. I'm really proud of doing that, because when I took this job, I thought to myself that I really wanted to have some other things I achieve over the same space of time, so I'm really pleased I've done that.

**Susie:** You're not short of adventures and challenges, you've just married for the first time (Peter Overton from *60 Minutes*) and obviously news and current affairs isn't too far away from your dinner table … How much has that changed you?

**Jessica Rowe:** Well, I love being married. I'm so happy. It almost leaves me speechless thinking about it, because when I was younger, I thought, 'I don't want to get married.'

My parents split up when I was young and I looked at them and thought I don't want to go down that path, no I'm not going to have children. And for a long time, I suppose through my mid-twenties, I was like 'No I don't want to be married and I can't imagine finding someone that I want to spend my life with,' and then I sort of came around and got to the point where I thought, 'No I really do want to find the love of my life.'

I met Peter and three years later we're married and I couldn't be happier and it's such a strange feeling because I knew being married would make me happy but I had no idea how happy it really would make me feel. It sounds a bit old fashioned but the sense of security, safety and stability that it brings to my life that he brings to my life is so comforting, it's wonderful! It's almost like I can finally breathe out (Jessica breathes out) and go he's there, he's with me, he'll look after me and I'll look after him too. But it's just such a lovely feeling to know there is someone who will walk the journey with you, who will be there with you.

**Susie:** Were you always tall, slim and drop dead gorgeous?

**Jessica Rowe:** When I was a teenager I had terrible acne, terrible skin and also into my early twenties I had terrible skin and that was awful. I would talk to people with my hands over my face thinking I could try and hide it and then I would go through phases where I would even try and turn them into beauty spots. But my skin really got to me. They found out it was to do with a hormone imbalance, so once investigated and treated properly it cleared. But I'm still paranoid about my skin because of the memory of how it did make me feel.

**Susie:** Where you a fussy eater as a child?

**Jessica Rowe:** No, no, Mum would cook us really healthy food, lots of fresh fruit and veg, and things like McDonald's or lollies were treats. They weren't in the cupboard; you couldn't just go and get them. They were for a special occasion, which I think was good, because we did learn healthy eating habits. We'd still be able to have junk food every now and then and lollies, but it was a treat, it wasn't something that you did every day.

**Susie:** You did some modelling before you started in television?

**Jessica Rowe:** I did do a little bit. I took a year off from my study in Bathurst, and did some modelling over the holidays, which led to me going to Germany for a six-week shoot that became a year and I am so pleased I did that. It got to me though and at the end of that year, I wanted to take another year off and travel but the uni said to me that I'd lose my place if I did, so I came back and finished my degree. Otherwise, who knows what I would be doing. But it was funny, the modelling, I was never very good at it. I was doing it at a time when it was big boobs and big blonde hair, all this sort of stuff, which isn't me – I've got no boobs and short hair (laughs) so it was kinda like the waif look hadn't arrived yet.

**Susie:** Do you have to watch your weight?

**Jessica Rowe:** Not in the sense of putting it on I don't. I'm really lucky, if anything I have to watch that I don't lose too much weight. I have always been slim but have found when I've been going through stressful times, or been working hard or not sleeping, I can get too thin, I think.

**Susie:** You engaged a personal trainer at times as well?

**Jessica Rowe:** I was very slim but I wanted to bulk up a bit, strengthen myself and be healthy. That started six years ago and I am still training with James Ardagna and he is the most lovely guy. What I like so much about him is when I first met him, he said 'What is it you want to do?' I said, 'I want to get fit, but also want to get a bit more muscly and a bit more bulky,' and he said, 'Okay, we'll do that,' and six years later he is still training me. I work-out twice a week; we lift weights, sometimes we'll do super sets and sometimes we have a strength phase. I'm really pleased, I've probably put on maybe 8 kilos since I started training, overall, with James. I'm really happy with that because I feel healthy, I feel strong and I've never thought of myself as a strong person, but to look at a whole lot of weights and think 'I can lift that, I can dead lift that' and to have guys at the gym going 'Hey, how do you lift that,' it's fantastic.

I love having muscly arms and shoulders and I always tease James and say 'I want to be like Ripley in *Alien,* you know how she has those fantastic arms' (laughs) and Linda in *Terminator* when she's doing all that (does the poses and laughs). That was kind of like my inspiration, that's when I'll be thinking 'Right, Ripley …'

**Susie:** You did cop your fair share of anorexia speculation in the press.

**Jessica Rowe:** Yeah, yeah. It was awful and it was all rubbish. From the outset, let me say it was rubbish, but to me it was so hurtful. It almost invited people to say 'Have you got an eating problem?

Why don't you eat up, what's wrong with you?' I would look at them and think I would never dream of saying to someone who was slightly overweight, 'Are you sure you want to eat that piece of cake?' or 'Are you exercising? Have you got an eating problem?' It was almost as if 'You're thin, you're fair game, so we can have a go at you' … and it's not fair, I found it really hurtful, especially seeing it wasn't true.

**Susie:** What's changed now in your routine? Did you ever run or exercise?

**Jessica Rowe:** No, I hate running (laughs). I hate it, if I went running I would lose too much weight and that's not what I want to do. So what I've been doing for the last six years has been the weight training, which I have found has worked very well for my body shape. And that's the key for people to find what works for them, because weight training might not be someone else's answer, they might prefer running or doing aerobics or yoga but for me I like weight training. I like what it does to my body and I also like the way it helps clear my mind of stress. I find it a real leveller to do that twice a week and if I don't I get a bit scratchy and more uptight, so I enjoy both the mental and physical benefits that it brings to me.

**Susie:** Of course there's the misconception that if you lift weights you are going to wind up with big muscles and looking like Arnold Schwarzenegger …

**Jessica Rowe:** Look at me, I'm not Arnie, not at all. It's not about that. I've got long limbs and the weight training just adds muscle and tone, and it's not giving me a big footballer's neck. I mean I joke with my trainer and go 'Is this the footballer's neck exercise?' (laughs) But no, it doesn't happen and if you choose the right sort of exercises it doesn't. Weight training builds your muscle, it's fantastic to have muscle.

**Susie:** So what eating plan do you live by? What do you eat for breakfast, lunch, dinner and snacks?

**Jessica Rowe:** It depends, I'm a healthy eater. I do have a sweet tooth, so I like to indulge that every now and then, but I think balance is important and I think when you start getting too

STILL HALF MY SIZE

preoccupied about what you can't eat and depriving yourself of things, then it can become an obsession and you fixate on it. I'm not into the savoury, I prefer the more sweet sort of things. For brekkie I'll eat toast, or muesli and yoghurt, cup of coffee. I love crumpets, I had that this morning, crumpets and honey. I go through phases. If I'm in here over lunchtime at work, I'll have a tuna sandwich, sometimes soup, whatever. I wish I was more organised and brought stuff in, but I'm never organised (laughs). And then for dinner sometimes I'll have pasta or chicken or seafood, it just depends. I like to have a glass of wine on the weekends and as I said, I have a sweet tooth, so love the occasional Cherry Ripe, pavlova, but I don't do it every night. I might have something sweet once a week or so.

**Susie:** I'm not hearing any red meat in there, is that right?

**Jessica Rowe:** That's a good point. I don't eat big bits of red meat, but I love sausages (laughs) and people say 'Don't you realise that's the worst type of meat?' I love bacon and pasta and that kind of thing. But I don't crave it.

**Susie:** Do you use food as a comfort or pig out or anything?

**Jessica Rowe:** I definitely use food, like if I have a Cherry Ripe or something like that I might be really craving something sweet. Often before my period I think, 'I need something sweet, I need a bit of a lift.'

**Susie:** Do you miss any meals?

**Jessica Rowe:** No way, that is the worst possible thing you can do. It is really important to eat your three meals, because if you skip breakfast you are starving by lunch, you eat too much of the wrong types of foods, it slows your metabolism down. Oh no way.

**Susie:** What about snacks? Do you eat between meals?

**Jessica Rowe:** Not really. Occasionally. I don't think I eat enough fruit, sometimes I think I should eat more fruit. That's what I should be eating between meals, but I don't. I might grab a yoghurt, but then sometimes I'll get a coffee, which isn't that good for me. Not a bad idea is a smoothie, sometimes I'll do that in the afternoon, when I feel my energy is starting to dip and normally I'd have a coffee and I think 'No, have a banana smoothie.' I get them to put an egg into it – you can't taste the egg, so you've got the protein and that's good because it fills you up and gives you an energy boost.

**Susie:** Do you have strong willpower?
**Jessica Rowe:** Yeah, I do.

**Susie:** Where does that come from?
**Jessica Rowe:** I think from my mum, she's such a brave, determined woman and I think from her.

**Susie:** But you're a brave, determined woman too. You and Peter did one of the most amazing stories I've ever seen on *60 Minutes* about mental illness and I congratulate you on it.
**Jessica Rowe:** I think, with mental illness it affects so many people. Mum has bipolar disorder and I have, over the years, spoken a lot about mental illness and getting rid of the stigma. I'd spoken a lot about it and so has Mum, but we'd never done it together in that way and also to have my new husband interviewing me and his new mother-in-law …

It is something that affects so many families and if Peter doing the story, first of all makes more people watch it but also brings home the point that he is a part of this family – look it happens here, we're getting on with life, life can be happy and positive – then it is a story worth telling. We decided if it made a difference to one person then it would be worthwhile, and we were overwhelmed by the response and that continues to reassure me and mean that it has had an impact on people.

**Susie:** Are you a procrastinator?
**Jessica Rowe:** I am sometimes, yes (laughs). I'm funny because some things I will do straight away and be focused on but other things I go, 'Nope, I can't be bothered.' For example, Pete and I went to Melbourne about a month ago and I still haven't unpacked my bag from Melbourne (laughs).

**Susie:** We've spoken about self-esteem issues with your skin, did that affect you, and obviously this is pre-marrying Peter, did that affect you going out with guys?

**Jessica Rowe:** Oh definitely. Definitely. I didn't feel attractive at all. I don't know if gloomy is the right word. I never felt I was one of the pretty girls at school or the ones that all the guys thought were terrific. I always felt awkward, unattractive and not confident.

**Susie:** Do you have any tips on overcoming mental obstacles when it comes to achieving aims and goals?

**Jessica Rowe:** I think you have to trust yourself and there are always people out there who will want to knock you down, criticise you. Don't listen to them, listen to yourself but also surround yourself with positive people, believe in what you can do.

Jess and Peter are now the proud parents of two gorgeous daughters; Allegra and Giselle. Jess is a three-time best-selling author. In January 2015, Jess was awarded an AM, a Member of the Order of Australia, in the Australia Day honours for her mental health advocacy. You can read more at jessicarowe.com.au

# CHAPTER 10

# SMOKE & MIRRORS

'While they're looking at the good bits, they're not looking at the bad bits.'
— ANNEMARIE ELELMAN

This was one of my mum's favourite sayings. To say she was a brilliant dressmaker and designer would be an understatement. Before I was born Mum worked for a couple of knitwear companies when she first came to Australia. Mum also worked in the wardrobe department at Artranza Studios when *Mission Impossible* star Peter Graves starred in a television series shot in Australia called *Whiplash*.

Money was scarce for us when we were growing up. Dad drove a truck for a boiling down works at Oxford Falls, picking up bones from all the butcher shops. Mum and Dad needed extra money so Dad converted the old laundry out the back of our place into a sewing room for Mum. When I'd come home from school I'd always hear the sound of her big industrial Singer sewing machine going before I'd rounded the corner to the backyard.

It was always wonderful to see what she had created and to watch the delight on the faces of the brides and their entourage when they all tried on their gowns. I'd get excited when I knew they were coming for their final fittings. Not only did I marvel at these gorgeous creations, but Mum always seemed to find time, and don't ask me how, to make dolls clothes from the leftover pieces of fabric as a treat for me.

Mum also made most of these amazing bridal gowns with detachable trains. Balls were really big back then, and everyone wore ball gowns so Mum would then help the brides dye their dresses after their big day to wear again.

One thing Mum hated doing, but it brought in extra cash, was alterations. She used to charge a guinea, which is one pound and one shilling (about $1.10 in decimal currency). The reason she despised it was because she had a few high society clients who wouldn't admit to the sales staff in the local fashion boutique what size they were so they'd intentionally buy a smaller size and bring it to Mum to alter. If there was not enough in the seams to let out, Mum would have to pick the entire outfit apart and literally remake it and then they'd argue that it should still only cost a guinea.

There's no doubt Mum gave me my passion for fashion but she also showed me how to highlight the 'good' bits and to conceal the 'bad' bits. Whether you're a size 10 or size 20, and remember I've been both, there's always a part or parts of us that we've never really been happy with, and no matter how much we exercise and eat correctly we can never physically change that part of us.

When I look at Elle Macpherson, I see how she deserves the title of 'The Body' because she is simply stunning and I can't see any flaws. But Elle has admitted in many interviews that her body is far from perfect. She cleverly won't admit what and where those imperfections are and she maintains that if we can't spot them then she's not going to point them out. While I'm sure Elle's imperfections would be assets on me, it's all about how we see ourselves, not how others see us.

While most of us can only dream of having Elle's body we can however learn a lot from her. We can all change people's perception of our size and shape by what we wear and the way we wear it. I hope you enjoy reading this chapter as much as I did interviewing internationally acclaimed dress designer Christopher Essex. I always affectionately called Christopher Essex my Frank Lloyd Wright of fashion because he's the best architect of a woman's body I've ever known.

Christopher created the majority of my early Logie outfits and not only has he created some amazingly stunning gowns, he has also managed to defy gravity as well! Despite the enormous public and media backlash I received when I wore that first, now infamous black and white Logie dress, which put me on my first worst dressed list and prompted journalist Julietta Jameson to brilliantly described me in one newspaper as looking like 'a herd of zebras rampaging down the red carpet', I was still thrilled with the results and I felt great in it. And believe it or not, Christopher made me look much slimmer than I really was underneath.

I've drawn on Christopher's expertise in this chapter to learn how to look our best regardless of what size is on the label of our clothes. Later in this chapter celebrity photographer Belinda Rolland details ways you can pose for photos to look slimmer. Belinda explains how simple it is to make a double chin seem to diminish just by the way we stand and hold our head.

## The mirror test

Time now to focus on your duco and upholstery and if both of these are well maintained then we can belie our chronological age and give the illusion that we've wound back the odometer. We can look and feel younger and if we look good, we feel good.

The first thing we need is to do is create a manual for our body so we understand what are the highlights and what would benefit more from being on low beam. The first step to ensure we look our best is to take that critical look at ourselves. This is best done in front of a full-length mirror and, if you can handle it, naked. If that's too traumatic do it in your underwear.

You need to assess your appearance and make a list of your strong and weak points. I suggest that you put your 'good points' down one side of the page and your 'not so good points' on the other. And if you're already thinking that your 'good points' list will be empty then I suggest that you add lack of self-confidence to your 'not so good' point list and aim to work on your self-esteem first.

I'm always reluctant to use the word 'bad' as we don't want to turn this into a negative experience. We are going for honesty, not soul destruction. It doesn't matter whether you start from your head down or your feet up – whatever way you find less daunting. I want you to systematically work your way through all your body parts and if you see them as an asset put them in the 'good' point list and what's not, goes on the other side.

Don't overlook a single feature from head to toe and make sure you take note if you have a dazzling smile and sparkling eyes. A great smile and eyes can give a positive impression around other people. What will emerge is your own personal blueprint that will show you what parts of your body you should be shining the spotlight on and what bits you should be keeping in the shadows.

'A woman's dress should be like a barbed wire fence
– serving its purpose without obstructing the view'.
– SOPHIA LOREN

# Christopher Essex interview

Christopher Essex grew up in a family and household where using a sewing machine was as common as watching television is today. In 1959, at the age of sixteen, Chris joined the original Mark Foy's department store as a machinist, making store display backdrops. As a result of his innate talent it wasn't long before he became principal machinist.

By the mid-1960s, Christopher was the main costume designer and maker for the majority of nightclubs and their shows in Sydney. Over the next ten years this involvement in the nightclub and entertainment industry expanded with his own boutiques stretching from Sydney to the Gold Coast, Hong Kong and London.

Christopher returned to Sydney in the mid-1970s for health reasons, eventually capturing the entire Sydney nightclub circuit again, including dressing the original and world famous Les Girls for ten years. Long before Christopher made my first Logies dress, I had the honour of working with him, hosting a series of spectacular TAFE fashion parades that he'd produced and coordinated. His talents were also showcased in the Star City Showroom when he designed and made all the costumes for the musical *Get Happy*. Christopher has also costumed many other live shows including *Red Hot & Rhonda, Private Lives, Lend Me a Tenor* and *Hot Shoe Shuffle*.

Christopher was always kept very busy creating divine gowns for special occasions, brides and the wedding party. With Christopher's tips you can then become a fashion illusionist when you master the art of camouflage. Just like a magician, it's all smoke and mirrors.

**Susie:** Everyone wants to look stylish. Do most people have a sense of style?

**Christopher Essex:** They do, but I think it's about comfort in your dress style and sense. I'm sure that you're born with it, but depending on the size of our wallet, you can sure buy it if you are bright enough to know. If you don't have it and you have a wallet that will accommodate it get a coordinator.

I think your sense of style can also be honed. Each one of us needs a Svengali who can guide you and help you hone your decisions about fashion and dress sense. Most of us need basic daywear that has an edge or is smart. Not all of us have the luxury of spending most evenings at cocktail parties and galas. I've noticed over the past few years that the younger generations look as if they belong to an army. They all look exactly the same, they speak the same dialogue, they wear the same things, they all look alike and this is because peer pressure is so strong these days. These fashions are not smart, they have become a uniform. The individual, and the sense of the individualistic, is falling by the wayside I sense.

And yet, to a degree, they emulate their pop divas, who look different year in and year out, especially during seasonal changes in the Northern Hemisphere. What we, the general public, don't realise is that they are all being styled by someone.

**Susie:** Should we wear what's fashionable or what suits us?

**Christopher Essex:** I think you should wear what suits you. Fashion can be the width of the leg of a trouser or the width of a lapel – basically that will stay in for a decade and you're pretty safe within that. But wear a skirt length that suits your leg and your body proportion; don't wear a miniskirt if you'd tell someone not to if they had the same body shape as you.

**Susie:** What is the ideal dress length?

**Christopher Essex:** I'll come back to it again. The ideal dress length is the one that suits you. And the only way to find this out is to explore. I suppose this is one area where it pays not to be too blinkered about fashion and try on things that you may not, initially, like.

I personally don't like mid-calf-length skirts; I find they tend to make legs look a little bowed, due to the shape of inner calf and ankle. They also make feet appear larger than they really are. With dress length I don't think there's a rule of thumb, but there is a certain area around the knee that is the most flattering and it varies from woman to woman. It could be at the base of knee, especially if you have a long knee to ankle; if you have that length in the calf it makes a big difference.

**Susie:** Who should we dress for?

**Christopher Essex:** Yourself. No question of it. If you satisfy yourself then you will satisfy those around you. Today, the emphasis seems to be on hot and sexy, but you know clothes are an inanimate object, you certainly can't say it's sexy because your knockers are hanging out. You can ooze sex appeal and be completely covered from head to toe because sex appeal is something that comes from within. Often the clothes are a catalyst that makes you feel hot or frumpy. So dress for yourself and dress in a way to make you feel the way you want to be perceived.

**Susie:** How can women look slimmer when they dress?

**Christopher Essex:** If you go out locally, anywhere that you live, have a look at what people are wearing. You'll find a lot of people who are larger than the average seem to dress in clothes that are too small for them to begin with, and which show little flare and style in cut or colour.

Tip number one: Make sure your clothes fit you. Clothes that are too tight make you look larger than you are.

Tip number two: Wear clothes that show others how you want to feel. Choose colours for the season as well. As warm as they can be in winter, leave the tracksuits for the gym.

Tip number three: Try wearing men's business shirts. Crisp, clean and ironed. Roll the sleeves up, and put the collar up as well. White or black for a change. Very smart and certainly slimming!

Tip number four: Don't wear pants with elastic waists. Wear clothes with a fixed size waistband so that you are aware of your body shape and weight changes.

**Susie:** What's the best skirt to wear for a woman with big hips?

**Christopher Essex:** The skirt must fall from the widest point of the hip. The material should have soft movement but not have any stretch.

**Susie:** And for a woman with a larger bust?

**Christopher Essex:** A very deep bust dart is the answer for clothes cut for women. This is also where a man's business shirt comes in handy – and can be very sexy as well. A white shirt or a white T-shirt under a shirt, I think it can give you a lovely crisp, very relaxed, comfortable in your clothing look, whilst you're losing weight.

**Susie:** Is that a key to being stylish, to highlight your good points and camouflage your not-so-good points?

**Christopher Essex:** The first thing is to know what your good points are. We all have them – we just have to honest with ourselves about them. I find it a strength to know how to apply make-up well. You can paint on a great face if you know the art of make-up. If you know how to handle your hair it's also a strength. But simply, as long as you look clean, and your hair looks clean and fresh, with healthy skin, those are things I find most important and lovely. With that said, what appeals to me may not appeal to the next person.

**Susie:** Are there any total no-no's in fashion?

**Christopher Essex:** Yes, there are just two rules. Don't choose a style or fashion that doesn't suit you or makes you uncomfortable. Go against either of these two rules and you are presenting yourself in an unflattering manner.

**Susie:** How important is underwear?

**Christopher Essex:** For a woman, very important depending on what she's wearing. I dress brides by the dozen and in certain dresses and fabrics you end up saying, 'Honey, you can't wear anything under that, you can't wear pants,' which is a strange thing. Well, I suppose not a strange thing to say to a bride, because she won't have them on for terribly long to begin with! Sometimes even a G-string can give you a line.

A well-fitted bra is also important because you won't look as big in the bust, and you won't get quilting across your back. I think you have to have an array of underwear that goes under various garments. Always have flesh coloured underwear to wear under white. Because there is such a variety of bras that are made for sporting, relaxing and evening, unfortunately you won't get one piece of underwear to do 24 hours.

**Susie:** Do posture and deportment play a part in showing your style?

**Christopher Essex:** Very much. Shoulders back. Shoulders back and tuck your ass in and go for it. Some of the younger girls today show a lack of deportment. I find it extraordinary how many times I have a gaggle of bridesmaids at the boutique and if they are on the sofa, their heads will be against the wall, they'll slide right down forward and their legs drift apart … you know like a teenage boy sort of thing. Behaving in a way to be seen as cool, relaxed and unfazed can be so unattractive.

**Susie:** What about fashion and posture?

**Christopher Essex:** Round shoulders are exceptionally difficult to deal with. Everything collapses, their bust sits lower, they're broad backed and narrow fronted. I think social skills and deportment should be part of your school syllabus.

**Susie:** What about accessories? And is the old adage, 'less is best' true anymore?

**Christopher Essex:** Are you talking about diamonds when you say that? If the accessories are real then more is more. But otherwise, less is definitely best. Understated lifts, overstated is tawdry.

**Susie:** What should an accessory do?

**Christopher Essex:** It should enhance whatever you're wearing. I don't think anything does it more than a shoe; the shoe can make or break a look. With women the two important things about them are the top and the bottom – head and feet. But to have a nice shoe and a lovely ankle and leg and a great head of hair, I think are the two greatest props a woman can have. They're the two accessories I think are most important: hair and ankle.

**Susie:** Any tips for someone with thick ankles?

**Christopher Essex:** I think pants are much more flattering very often than anything else.

**Susie:** What about colours? Are we a certain colour? We hear about this, 'you're a summer, you're a winter' etcetera.

**Christopher Essex:** I don't know whether all of that's real; I suppose there's an element of truth in it. But I think you can put on a colour and suddenly you feel well, you feel happy without being aware that the colour is the catalyst. And you can feel vibrant and alive and you can put on another colour and think 'Oh I feel dreary as bum today, what is it?'

Colour lifts you, you can put it on and it absolutely transports you. Your body and hair combine differently in summer and winter, even if you don't change hair colour. Our skin colour changes between summer and winter, whether we sunbathe during summer or not.

But, I think you have to go in and explore colours. Even if you just go into your local fabric shop and throw a piece of colour across you. There are some tips for a Western culture though. Anyone with olive skin for example should steer clear of limes and yellows because they can make you think 'Ohhh God, I look ill.' Purple is another interesting colour – especially if you're an emperor or a Queen! It can work well with many age groups and body shapes. It's a spectrum of colour I hear most people call purple, anything under that spectrum of colour. But it's a very pretty shade, all those lavenders, mauves, wisterias, all those colours, yet you don't see too much of it worn.

When people ask, 'What are the new fashion colours?' my response is usually 'It doesn't matter because if it's a colour that doesn't suit you, you won't wear it. Just wear what makes you look sensational.'

**Susie:** Is it important to get the right tone of colour?

**Christopher Essex:** Oh yes, take brown for example. It can be as dreary as bum, but you can get wonderful shades of brown from gold toffee tones, which are lovely, to that old mission brown, which you wouldn't want for free.

**Susie:** What do you recommend for a short and stocky body shape?

**Christopher Essex:** Depends upon the personality of the person. If they are comfortable with their body shape I find that their dress sense is pretty on the mark. I don't need to do much for these people except maybe to try to get them to explore a little more. If they appear to be a little uneasy about their body shape I tend to go overboard a bit and show them a whole new side to themselves.

Once, for an entertainer who is short and stocky, I made an outfit that was pure clotted cream with a cream embroidered spangly tabard that went over the top of it. It was such a shock reaction when she saw it, and when she put it on it was absolutely transforming, her whole persona changed. I made her something that she would never have thought of.

She was an entertainer so she needed to have a statement. I think those of us who aren't entertainers can still make great statements. You just have to have the chutzpah and the bravado to be willing to try new things occasionally. The change in style brought out a side of her that had always been there but hidden by her camouflage clothes.

**Susie:** For someone who is short and a bit stocky, would a dress and a jacket be better than a skirt and a jacket?

**Christopher Essex:** I think problem figures are usually better dealt with in pieces, because you can break the figure at the top hip, lower hip, mid-thigh, you can lower it and break it up or whatever. So dresses are a bit more difficult for this sort of thing. Dresses present problems that skirts don't when sitting for example. When buying clothes, make sure you sit in them, worry about standing in them, but sit in them as well. It's very important to sit in new clothes, because you spend a lot of time sitting.

If you start plucking and tugging at your clothes, it'll only draw the eye to that bit you are plucking and tugging at.

**Susie:** What if you are really tall?

**Christopher Essex:** The same thing applies, you can wear wonderful statements or you can try and hide. More than anything whether you're tall or short, you have to get the proportions right between length and the taper of legs and sleeves. Buying clothes off the rack is made for middle of the road, so if you're short you need to find a good tailor to make the alterations you'll need. And make sure you don't just take up or let down the cuff of the pants; taper the leg to get the proportion back because if you take it up six inches the mid-thigh will be at your knee, so the proportion between length and width is wrong. The same thing if you are tall. Check if there is allowance in the cuff to let it down, you can always let it down and have a facing put on it.

Sleeve lengths are the same as well. Short cuffs emphasise height or growing out of clothes, long cuffs look buffoonish. So if it sits above the ankle or the wrist, you may look and feel ungainly.

**Susie:** What about pleated skirts?

**Christopher Essex:** Pleats are fine if they are not disturbed. The only caution is for women who may be broad of hip. Only wear pleats that are stitched in from the waist. If they are sewn in, down to lower hip, then they will fall undisturbed from lower hip. If they are pleated into the waistband they will stretch and the fall will be destroyed and you'll have a lot of bulk.

**Susie:** We had big padded shoulders in the eighties and I've noticed quite a number of fashion items today are creeping back into smaller shoulder pads. Do they have a purpose? Are they important?

**Christopher Essex:** They are absolutely very important. Most women have very narrow sloping shoulders, it isn't the width of the shoulder, it's the elevation. You can still wear shoulder pads in so many things and just to give you that extra height in the shoulder line, not widen the shoulder, elevate the shoulder.

Sensible use of shoulder pads makes your clothes fall better. They take that creasing away from shoulder to armpit line, which makes any fashion look sad. Buy a pair of very good shoulder pads that are moulded and they'll cap your shoulder. Put them under your bra strap and they'll sit there undetected totally, but will give you a much crisper look.

**Susie:** What's happened to the waist?

**Christopher Essex:** It's disappeared as a fashion point. The old 36, 25, 36 isn't around anymore. Girls are much thicker through the waist than they ever used to be so I don't think many people worry about the waist today. Modern generations have grown up with hipsters and they don't think of them as hipster, they've lowered their waist to that area. A waist can be a wonderful area depending entirely on what you are wearing. Someone who's got a great figure and emphasises a waist can look wonderful, but we don't live in an era of waistlines, we really don't.

**Susie:** What about stripes?

**Christopher Essex:** Stripes will accentuate any lumps and bumps you have, as will the material. Stretchy, stripy clothes will make any lumps and bumps appear much larger than they really are. On some they can look fabulous because they are so bold. I think it all depends on the fit of the garment more than anything.

**Susie:** Do you think we get to an age where we can't wear certain fashion?

**Christopher Essex:** You can't wear young, young, young stuff when you've had a few summers under your belt. But why would you want to? You move on, you are a different person, you're not that person anymore and if you are aware of it, your figure changes, your face changes, your colouring changes. By that stage you should be comfortable with who you are and develop your style.

**Susie:** Are there any other tips you can give me on developing a style?

**Christopher Essex:** For a woman there are no restrictions except the restrictions she puts on herself. I dress a lot of women who are very stylish and I'm only one component in their world. I admire the style they have, I love watching a woman and the unaware things she will do: how she will handle her hair, how she goes through a fitting of her clothes, how she sits, how she walks, those things, I think, are absolutely fascinating.

I admire a lot of the women I make stuff for, for their individuality, and they are all women who are on the other side of 40, 50 or 60. I have two women in their eighties, who are smart as paint, absolutely smart as paint, I think 'Aren't you fabulous, fabulous.' Not anything over the top, not mutton dressed as lamb, just innately stylish and comfortable in themselves and have been comfortable for a long, long time.

**Susie:** What would be the key things you need in your wardrobe? If you were planning to put a wardrobe together, given that in most cases dollars are always the problem, what are some of the must-haves in your wardrobe?

**Christopher Essex:** Well, I think a woman always needs about five pairs of shoes, your absolute minimum. If you were starting with nothing, walked in barefoot, women need many more shoes than a man ever does.

A couple of very good bags, something in a taupe and a black – good bags of a medium, moderate size, not great big shopping jobs. A couple of good shirts, shirts are always a great thing for women. A couple of good T-shirts. A great jacket, probably something that's a little bit longer rather than short that can be worn with pants. A good pair of pants, a good pair of jeans. Don't worry about if you can't even find something that's cut to the waist, but just that it fit you well, gives you a good arse and leg line and don't have any bits rolling over the top of it.

Maybe one good shaped dress, you only have to go to the outlets and you can find something in a basic, neutral colour, enough to go with your few pieces. You can then add vibrancy maybe with a marvellous scarf or a flower or a T-shirt, beads. But get your basics right.

**Susie:** What about men? Are there some tips on how they can look stylish and slimmer? Let's start with trouser length …

**Christopher Essex:** Trousers must always break on the arch of the shoe. I also recommend longer socks; ones that pull up almost to the knee. I think it's very unsavoury when a man sits down and pulls his trousers up and you see shoe, socks, skin, pants; it's the same as a woman wearing knee-highs under a skirt.

**Susie:** What about the suit? Double-breasted versus single-breasted?

**Christopher Essex:** I like all of them. I like a two-button, three-button suit, I like a double-breasted. I think they have a totally different feeling. I'm not personally fond of suits that button almost to the throat, they always remind me of Beatlemania – we're too old for that!

**Susie:** Tie length. Are there rules for the length of the front piece of a tie?

**Christopher Essex:** The Duke of Windsor used to wear the front of his tie very long so that it appeared below his jacket. He made it a fashion statement. It was all wrong but it was his statement and he carried it off. The bottom of the front piece of a tie should just touch the belt of the trousers, maybe go a little beyond but not much. That's the general rule.

**Susie:** Men and tummies – any suggestions?

**Christopher Essex:** The same rules apply – make sure you wear clothes of the right size. They fall correctly and look crisp and clean. If you look back at the movies and see Sydney Greenstreet, who was an enormously big man, beautifully tailored, he was tailored for his movies obviously. With jacket types, you can wear all of them as long as they fit you now, not fit you as you were ten years ago.

**Susie:** And what about colours and patterns for men?

**Christopher Essex:** Well, most men's stuff isn't coloured or patterned, unfortunately. If you can find it try using the same colour rules as apply for women. It's just so difficult to find coloured and patterned clothes for men in Australia.

**Susie:** In summing up, what would be your best tip to give a woman to improve the way she thinks of herself?

**Christopher Essex:** Look good and feel good. Feel good and look even better. Step back from the crowd. You can't be everyone. You can't be all things to all people. If you're true to yourself and you find something and you are absolutely happy in, then something must be right about it. If you have reservations, then there's obviously something wrong, find out what's wrong about it. Explore things – just because it's the local momentary fashion that really shouldn't come into it at all. But there are certain things you can put on and you know, well you have to know they are right, you put them on and feel good. When you feel good in particular clothes try and work out why.

Sadly, Christopher Essex succumbed to a second bout of cancer in 2006 at only 61. I still have all his amazing creations, they are works of art and I hope the Powerhouse Museum will want them for posterity. Wollongong dressmaker and designer Peter Bartlett has been creating my Logie outfits since 2008.

## Shying away from photos

As you'll see from some of the photos I've included in this book, the bigger I became the more ways I'd find to try and hide behind other people to make it look like I was smaller.

Many people shy away from cameras altogether, in fact one of the hardest tasks for Weight Watchers is to gather 'before' shots of the finalists in their annual Healthy Life Awards. This is a real tragedy because you then realise there's no recorded history or images for family to remember you by.

On my afternoon show on Radio 2GB I always looked forward to a visit from Belinda Rolland, who is a very well regarded celebrity photographer. Belinda would pop into the studio and fill us in on all the A-list events; who attended, what they wore and how they looked. At the end of all the fun celebrity news, Belinda would leave us with a tip on how to look your best in a photograph. She's included all those and lots, lots more in this interview.

# Belinda Rolland interview

**Susie:** Please start with the Belinda Rolland story.

**Belinda Rolland:** It all started when I moved to Sydney [from Brisbane] with my girlfriend at the time. She was pursuing her career in photography and I ended up working as her assistant for about a year and a half. I was on a photo shoot with her one day and was asked by a magazine if I'd like to shoot the socials. I jumped at the chance and it started from there.

I just got more and more into it and worked solidly and picked up some of Sydney's biggest PR jobs. I've officially photographed the AFI Awards, the Logies, Tropfest and now I do big events, PR, product launches, lots of film premieres and red carpets, perfume launches and of course the magazine work. It has snowballed, literally, to the point sometimes that I'm so busy I need three of me. But I can't complain, it's a great thing working for yourself and to be thought of as successful at it.

**Susie:** Who are some celebrities you have photographed on the red carpet?

**Belinda Rolland:** Oh some of the world's biggest. Nicole Kidman, Russell Crowe, Cate Blanchett, Rachel Griffiths … these are some of the Aussie ones. The biggest names that have come into Sydney – Pierce Brosnan, Jodie Foster, John Travolta, Keanu Reeves – gosh, the list is endless; anyone that's ever had a film premiere in Sydney and that's come out here to do it like the girls from *Charlie's Angels* – Drew Barrymore, Lucy Liu and Cameron Diaz – celebrity musicians and lots of actors, directors. There are thousands; I can't even begin to tell you. I've taken hundreds and thousands of photographs.

**Susie:** Do overweight people sometimes shy away from having their photo taken?

**Belinda Rolland:** Yes some do; and that's not just celebrities but people at parties. If they're larger women or men they're not as happy about having their photo taken, because they are very conscious of their weight and how they look or how they are going to be perceived in a photograph in a magazine.

**Susie:** Do you have tips on how to look slimmer in photos?

**Belinda Rolland:** Absolutely! There's an art to it. I get women or men if they are slightly overweight not to stand front on [to the camera], not to face me front on but to turn slightly on their side. It takes away the width. Looking at them front on makes them look as large as they are. If they turn to their side, you're only getting a profile so you're definitely taking away a few pounds. The end result of that is people don't look anywhere near as big as they may be and a lot of woman have walked away thinking that's how I'll deal with photos.

You can also sit down. I love taking shots of people sitting down because it gives you a whole different aspect and you're concentrating then on only getting a half-body shot. I like to do it because you can get people to lean forward: this gives them a nice neckline and cleavage and therefore you're not seeing so much of the stomach and the legs because you're doing the upper torso.

Sit on the edge of the seat, sit forward and put your hands in the shot. Make sure you lean forward into the shot and the top part of your torso and your face become the main frame of the photograph. Always sit forward not back. Maybe cross your legs and lean forward slightly from the hips.

**Susie:** For standing shots, what should you do with your feet?

**Belinda Rolland:** Well I think every woman should take a good look at how models stand; they're fantastic. Don't stand with your feet apart as if you're a builder or you've just gotten off a horse. You want to stand with one foot slightly forward and one foot slightly back and maybe have one foot with the toes pointing out. And I tell people to put their hands on their hips as it gives you a bit more shape. It's that classic model look; maybe the right foot forward, the other one behind about 30 centimetres or so, it gives your legs and outfit a much better shape.

**Susie:** Once you have your feet right, then you twist your body?

**Belinda Rolland:** Turn to your side, twist your upper body forward and if you're standing front on then twist your body to the side. Gives your outfit and your body different looks.

**Susie:** Should you practise in front of a mirror?

**Belinda Rolland:** I think it's a great idea, especially if you're wearing a dress that's got a great big split up it or something like that and you want to show off a bit of leg, definitely. Standing in front of a mirror before you go out and posing to see how best your outfit sits on you is one of my favourite tips.

**Susie:** Is that the key to highlight the good points that you feel you've got and display those in a photograph?

**Belinda Rolland:** Yes I think it's important, I really do. If you like the way you look or if you're pretty happy with an outfit you're wearing or your hair. I think you need to look at yourself and practise all the positions you can in front of a full-length mirror if you're going to walk a red carpet, or just make an entrance to a dinner party.

**Susie:** How can we look slimmer in our arms?

**Belinda Rolland:** Bend your arms. So many people stand in a picture with their arms straight by their side like they should be in a school photo and it's boring. If you want to look good in a picture, at least put one hand on your hip or both hands on your hip, it gets your hands into the photo, because if the photo gets chopped then you lose your arms and hands. If you've got a hat, put your hand on your hat holding the brim, it brings your hands into the shot.

**Susie:** How should we position our head?

**Belinda Rolland:** The head should always be slightly tilted forward from the neck, so put your neck out a little bit. Don't put your nose up so we shoot a shot up your nose! Just pop your neck out ever so slightly and it stops double chins and it makes your face almost the feature of the photograph.

**Susie:** Bending from the waist, what does that do?

**Belinda Rolland:** Yes. Lean forward from the waist. If the photographer wants to use a half-body shot, it ends up making your upper body the foremost part of the photograph. It makes a great shot.

**Susie:** Is it important to smile?

**Belinda Rolland:** If you don't smile it doesn't look like a social shot, it looks like you're having a bad time so why bother being there? Show your teeth if you've got nice teeth. I suppose if you've got crooked teeth, or you don't like your smile, try to smile but maybe don't show your teeth. Practise in a mirror until you find a smile you like.

**Susie:** What if you're in a group shot? How should you stand to look slimmer?

**Belinda Rolland:** In a group shot stand side on, not all facing the camera. This again reduces the size of the hips and things like that.

**Susie:** What if we feel conscious about a big nose?

**Belinda Rolland:** If you've got a big nose steer clear of doing profile shots. Look directly at the camera; don't turn your head left or right. If you were looking at someone with a large nose you wouldn't notice it being as large if they were looking straight on.

**Susie:** What sort of clothes photograph well?

**Belinda Rolland:** Colour photographs well. Stripes and checks and spots are not good for photography. But of course you can't stop people wearing those fashions and black is just boring photographically. Floral is fine, I don't know what it is about stripes, checks and spots … they just aren't good to photograph, they're too busy.

**Susie:** What mistakes do people make when they pose for photos?

**Belinda Rolland:** From experience I'd say we've covered most of the problem areas, don't face the camera, stand side on, keeping your legs together, lean forward from the waist, just pop the neck forward a little, and get your hands into the picture. But the most important tip is to have a smile that you're comfortable with – all too often I see very cheesy smiles.

# Susie's tips to combat negative body image

- Develop good posture and you will look confident

- Stand tall, sit tall, keep your chin up and shoulders back

- Identify your strengths and build on them

- Don't be too critical of yourself or dwell on the negatives

- Accept yourself – you can't overcome genetics

- Highlight your assets

- Improve your conversation skills

- SMILE!

# Self-esteem tips from celebrity lips

I hope next time someone offers to take your photo, rather than shying away you will try some of Belinda's tips instead and see if you like the results. You can take comfort in the fact that you and I aren't the only ones who are not totally happy with ourselves; every one of my celebrity interviewees found it easy to identify their good and not so good points. Here's an insight into what my contributors think about their own self-esteem. They also unveil whom they'd most like to resemble in looks, given the choice, and also what qualities they find appealing and unappealing in others.

**Susie:** If you could look like anybody in the world, living or dead, who would it be?

**Jeff Fenech:** I've been pretty lucky. Money and success make you look as good as anybody. But, if forced, I suppose Brad Pitt. It wouldn't be bad sitting on the beach or sitting in a restaurant, looking like him.

**Phebe Irwin:** Figure wise, Raquel Welch, but also I look at Magda Szubanski or Kirstie Alley and think good on you for being who you are.

**Trevor Hendy:** Oh when I was younger I just loved Elvis Presley. I don't know why.

**John Maclean:** Me. Because I am me. I can't worry about anybody else. I am who I am and that's a nice place to be.

**Dave Gorr:** I look at my body type and I couldn't possibly be a Brad Pitt because I'm too chunky. I'm not tall enough to be Arnold Schwarzenegger but I might be someone like a Sylvester Stallone type body.

**Sandra Sully:** Despite being a Pisces I am not a dreamer and more of a realist so I guess I accept who and what I am. I admire many but focus on being the best that I can be.

**Wayne Pearce:** I suppose it would be Brad Pitt, because he's got a head that hasn't been all bashed around, like me.

**Tara Moss:** Oh Angelina Jolie by a long shot. I think everyone either wants to look like her, be her, or be with her. She's a goddess. I love her.

**Shelley Taylor-Smith:** Me. Shelley Taylor-Smith. There's only one Shelley Taylor-Smith and I know this girl.

**Fran Macpherson:** I think Michelle Pfeiffer or Meg Ryan. I find both those women strong, so it's not wholly their looks.

**Jessica Rowe:** I'm happy with myself, I really am. Occasionally I think I'd love to have boobs and be a bit more curvy. But I'm happy in my own skin.

**Susie:** What do you find attracts you to someone?

**Sandra Sully:** Good looks are always a great start, but not the most important. I like integrity, a good heart and a good smile.

**Wayne Pearce:** I think someone that oozes energy, looks like they've got a bit of life about them.

**Tara Moss:** Humour, honesty, a good heart.

**Fran Macpherson:** A pulse! The eyes do it for me. And the mind. Smart is definitely sexy, a sense of style, good humour, confidence and clean fingernails. Height, I like tall men. I don't mind if a man has a bit of padding, can't have too much though. When they're with me they usually end up quite lean because I make them get up in the morning and run!

**Wayne Pearce:** You look around and you see some women carrying a little bit of weight and they look quite sexy.

**John Maclean:** I'm attracted to someone who's comfortable to be in their own skin and to be comfortable with who they are and to love who they are. That's a huge attraction because they say well this is me and I'm not going to pretend to be anyone else because I'm not.

**Jessica Rowe:** Of course, there's the physical attraction. It's kind of the vibe; an energy or some sort of connection. And different men, different things, a physical connection or there might be more of an intellectual connection.

**Phebe Irwin:** The eyes and the lips. The face. I know some people who are very out of shape but they've got lovely, lovely faces.

**Susie:** Do you think you feel less attractive to the opposite sex when you are overweight?

**Fran Macpherson:** Generally but it depends who you're with. An acquaintance of mine, whom I've known for many years, only ever has big girlfriends, I mean really big, but that's what he likes. I went out with a man for a while, who told me I was too skinny, because he liked big girls. Had to love him!

**Trevor Hendy:** No I have been before but I think once again its back to the person. You know it's funny with Jo my partner she's absolutely gorgeous and she's got an incredible body and she doesn't do anything to maintain it. Recently she felt she'd put on a bit of weight. I don't see that I just look at her and go you're incredible. You're beautiful. She still has trouble believing me I think.

**Jessica Rowe:** I don't know about attracted to someone's size, to me it's the overall package, so size isn't that important by itself.

**Dave Gorr:** I've been with both. I guess it would depend on how overweight. I've been with a couple of girls that were largish and they were sexy girls. But sexy is different.

**Phebe Irwin:** It's a confidence thing. I think that has a lot to do with it.

**Susie:** Who's a famous person you find attractive?

**Jeff Fenech:** I love Rachel Hunter. I mean Julia Roberts is absolutely beautiful, but I love Rachel Hunter, because she's not thin, thin, thin. I think she's absolutely gorgeous.

**Trevor Hendy:** At the moment I think it's Kate Beckinsale.

**Sandra Sully:** Well I could certainly look at Brad Pitt most weeknights, but, then again, who couldn't? There are lots of interesting, fascinating people. Looks fade. The heart and head is where it's at.

**Wayne Pearce:** Rachel Hunter.

**Fran Macpherson:** I do love Richard Gere, no matter if he is playing a goodie or a baddie. We have some really sexy local actors and I do find I am very attracted to Andrew Denton, because of his brain. I used to be extremely attracted to Clive Robertson also because of his brain. Smart turns me on.

**Shelley Taylor-Smith:** The sexiest man I reckon is George Clooney.

**Jessica Rowe:** Just behind my husband of course, is Hugh Jackman. I think he is hot; he is divine.

# CHAPTER 11

# ADD SEX AND DOUBLE YOUR RESULTS

'Self-esteem can't be measured in kilograms.
And when Cupid shoots his arrows, he aims for the heart, not the hips.'

— LIBBI GORR

No doubt I have your undivided attention, just from the title! Did you immediately turn to this chapter and read it first? Don't be embarrassed; it's something I would do too! If you were hoping this final chapter would be a kiss and tell all about my sex life, I'm sorry to disappoint you. I've made a few confessions in the previous chapters about a lot of my life but when it comes to sex I'm 'The Vault'. It's not something I broadcast or brag about and sex is certainly an area where people can be very judgmental. Even in today's supposed sexual equality, if a man is sexually active with a few partners he's considered a bit of a stud but a woman in the same position is more often regarded as a bit of a slut.

Whatever labels we put on those who are getting lots of sex, it would appear that they are in the minority. While most people will jokingly wish they were living their lives like an episode of *Sex and the City,* they're more likely to tell you it's the opposite and that they're actually not getting enough sex.

Does sex rate highly in your mind? I don't know if you've noticed it, or maybe it's just the company I keep, but sex doesn't ever seem to be very far away from a lot of social conversations. The question of where sex rates came up over a few drinks with some friends recently and one of the guys said, 'If sex doesn't come first on my list, it's at least ahead of what's in second spot!' We all laughed but everyone agreed that sex was, without a doubt, the best sensation on earth.

Dr Rosie King told me that Dr David Weeks, a consultant neuropsychologist at the Royal Edinburgh Hospital, even goes as far as saying, 'Pleasure derived from sex is a crucial factor in preserving youth.' And while all research is open to interpretation and people do lie, especially about sex, Dr Weeks came up with his 'elixir of youth' claim after interviewing more than 3500 people aged 18 to 102 in Britain, Europe and the US over ten years. His study found that couples who have sex at least three times a week look more than ten years younger than the 'average adult' who has sex twice a week.

It started me thinking that if something felt this good then surely it had to be good for you as well. I decided the best person to have a long chat with about this very subject is the ever-inspiring Dr Rosie King.

Dr Rosie is a doctor with a difference. A sex therapist and sex educator, she has helped thousands of men and women achieve greater happiness and health through her counselling practice and her appearance on television and radio and articles in health magazines. As always, she's full of good news and insightful information. Not only has Dr Rosie shared her sexpertise, Dr Gary Aaron has some tips on increasing our libido and I pose a few sexy questions to our celebrities and their fun responses are included as well.

# Dr Rosie King interview

**Susie:** How much sex is enough?

**Dr Rosie:** Sex is like salaries. Everyone thinks that everybody else is getting more than them. The way we carry on about 'getting enough' in the bedroom, you'd think that sex was some kind of competitive sport with a gold medal for the couple with the top sexual score. The recent Men's Sexual Habits Survey by Pfizer found that average sexual frequency in men and women aged 40 to 69 was between five to eight times per month, or about once or twice a week. Similar findings are reflected in other studies. Yet these 'average' figures can be misleading because they don't reflect the wide range of sexual activity. Some couples might need sexual intercourse five times a week to feel satisfied while others might be content with once a month or less.

**Susie:** How does sex stack up compared to other activities in burning kilojoules?

**Dr Rosie:** Sexual intercourse is an aerobic activity that burns up the same number of kilojoules as briskly climbing several flights of stairs. I've prepared a chart for my book *Sex Unlimited* (Random House) and you can see how sex compares to other exercises in energy consumption (see Appendix I). It's about the same as doing light housework but sex is definitely much more fun.

In fact the energy used up by sex is not very much at all, not your bread and butter sex. It's probably different if you're hanging from the chandeliers. But even fairly low-key lovemaking once a week will burn more than 10,000 kilojoules a year. And the more turned on we become, the more we tighten up the large muscles of the abdomen, thighs, buttocks, calves and even the face. This helps arousal and triggers sexual climax – and provides highly enjoyable isometric exercise.

**Susie:** What are some of the reasons sex is good for us?

**Dr Rosie:** Here are ten top reasons I can think of right away.

1. It helps us live longer. Research suggests sex lengthens your lifespan because it provides an abundance of skin-on-skin

contact. Sex is a specialised form of touching and touch is known to increase the secretion of substances that help us live longer.

2. An orgasm can help to relieve premenstrual tension and period pain as well. Most men don't need to be convinced that a regular sex life is good for them, however, it's men over the age of 40 that need regular sex to avoid congestion of the prostate. Build-up of fluid in the prostate due to infrequent orgasm can cause significant discomfort during ejaculation. The cure is simple, more orgasms.

3. Sex boosts self-esteem.

4. Raises oestrogen levels in women, which helps to keep female genitals moist and healthy.

5. Gets us to sleep. There is no better way to relax and get off to sleep than making love. That is because of endorphins, which are released from the brain after orgasm. They are feel-good chemicals and they create feelings of wellbeing and relaxation.

6. Gives a mini work-out. In men and women, sexual thoughts and acts increase testosterone levels, which not only enhance sexual desire but also increase the ratio of lean muscle to body fat. So if you want a great body, have more sex. And you can lie down while you do it!

7. Stress buster. Because sex is so relaxing it is wonderful for stress busting.

8. It improves our relationships too. Oxytocin is another chemical that is involved in sexual arousal and oxytocin is known as the cuddle chemical. When you are in a situation with another person where there is a lot of oxytocin in your system, you will feel emotionally bonded to them. In a long-term relationship, regular loving sex can act as both a glue and lubricant. It's a glue because it binds a couple together and a lubricant because when sex is good it helps to smooth over the rough edges of everyday life.

9. Sex is a great painkiller. Endorphins, the body's natural painkillers, are released from the brain after climax, flooding us with feelings of relaxation and wellbeing, as well as relieving pain. Sex can relieve a headache, sore neck or the pain of

arthritis because when we're turned on our pain threshold goes up.

10.   Sex is good for the pelvic floor. During sexual arousal the pelvic floor muscles tense and lift up, then contract firmly and rhythmically during orgasm in both sexes. Regular sexual activity helps to keep the pelvic floor muscles toned and terrific.

Most women are aware of the importance of pelvic floor fitness. If the pelvic floor is weak, partners will complain of loss of sexual feeling and women can suffer from problems such as stress, incontinence and prolapse of the pelvic organs.

**Susie:** Is regular masturbation healthy?

**Dr Rosie:** Woody Allen said, 'Don't knock masturbation. It's sex with someone I love.' Masturbation is normal; it's a powerful way for individuals to learn about their own sexuality so they can transmit this information to their partner.

Babies reach for their genitals and pleasure themselves as soon as they have the hand coordination to do so. Many young men and women experience their first orgasms through self-pleasuring. There's an old joke that claims 99 per cent of men masturbate and the other one per cent lie.

As long as it isn't interfering with your sexual relationship with your partner, self-pleasuring does have a role to play in relationships. And it is certainly a legitimate way to keep the sexual wheels turning when you're not in a relationship with a partner. However, if you have moral or religious beliefs that dictate that masturbation is wrong, your views should be respected.

**Susie:** What happens if one partner has a higher sex drive?

**Dr Rosie:** Well it's not if one partner has a higher sex drive. Most couples find that their sexual appetites differ. For some the difference in libidos is small; for others the gap between their levels of sexual desire is big enough to drive a truck through! A difference in libidos is known as desire discrepancy or DD. DD is the most common sexual difficulty experienced by couples. However it is not a sexual dysfunction or an abnormality. A pair of perfectly matched sex drives is as rare as hens' teeth. DD is not only normal; it is inevitable in long-term relationships. During the wonderful infatuation phase, when you are first courting, you can't keep your hands off each other and you are in bed every opportunity you can get. But those days of heady romance can't and don't last forever. At some point the love boat crashes against the shores of everyday life and differences in libido emerge.

If you think about it, we all have different needs. We have different needs for sleep, food, heat. Often when you are in a relationship with someone, opposites attract. Often a person who likes to go to sleep early will pair up with someone who likes to go to sleep late. The lark marries the owl. Relationships don't usually fail because one person likes to stay up late and the other one likes to get up early. But when it comes to sex there is a lot of angst and unhappiness because people have an expectation that they should have perfectly matched sex drives.

**Susie:** What could be some of the reasons for a decrease in libido?
**Dr Rosie:** Loss of sexual desire from time to time is normal.
If either partner in a relationship has lost their libido altogether they need a check-up with their GP to exclude physical and hormonal problems or depression.

Avoiding sex with a partner is frequently a reaction to criticism or hostility, either in or out of the bedroom or both. If it isn't temporary and it's been months or years since you felt any real desire, then I can understand how a partner's patience runs out.

These are my top reasons why your libido can drop into low gear.

1. Too tired. A tired woman is not a sexy woman. If your sex life has gone from horny to yawny, establish a healthy routine. Ensure a good night's sleep. Avoid caffeine in the evening; try a calming cup of chamomile instead. And get rid of the TV in the bedroom. Use your bed only for sleeping and sex.

2. Hormone havoc. Some women lose interest in sex in the second half of their cycle. If this is the case, or you suffer from PMS, take a magnesium supplement plus vitamin B complex throughout the month. Avoid foods containing

refined sugars and flour, and follow a low-fat diet with plenty of fresh fruit and vegies. Caffeine, nicotine and alcohol can aggravate PMS. Exercising can help.

3. Feeling low. When you're feeling depressed you couldn't care less about sex. The herb St John's wort can be useful for relieving anxiety and depression. And it has been estimated that half of all depression cases can be helped through some form of regular exercise.

4. Pill popping. Prescription medication can adversely affect sex drive. Some women notice that their interest in sex plummets when they start taking the pill, so a change in brand might be necessary. Antidepressant medication, tranquillisers, appetite suppressants, blood pressure medication, steroids, radiotherapy, chemotherapy and hormone therapy are among the drugs that can turn you off sex.

5. Stressed out. Sex and stress don't mix. To counter stress, say 'no' more often. Laugh. Spoil yourself. Take regular breaks. Practise yoga or some other stilling activity each day.

And finally, any problems with your relationship need to be addressed. Sometimes counselling will be necessary; sometimes it's just a matter of education and busting some myths about how sex should be. Some problems run deeper, particularly if there has been some history of untoward sexual experience like childhood sexual abuse or some sort of sexual assault. If these tips don't help see your GP for advice.

**Susie:** Love and lust, do they need to go hand in glove for a relationship to last?

**Dr Rosie:** There are three phases to a relationship. The first phase is pure physical attraction. You might think you love his mind, his ideas and his dreams for the future but in reality you are captured by his smile or the way he walks. It can't be love because you usually know very little about each other in the attraction phase.

The second phase is infatuation. It's known as the 'limerence'. It's that time when you are on your best behaviour, making a huge effort to appear 'perfect' to your lover. You both can't bear to be apart. It's a period of intense romantic feelings fuelled by a potent chemical cocktail swirling around in our systems. We feel as if we are madly in love because we are awash with hormones such as adrenaline, dopamine, phenylethylamine (PEA) and serotonin, which cause a state of ecstasy. Limerence is more lust than love.

The third phase is attachment. This is when we can really start to be ourselves around our partner and differences in needs and desires can emerge and conflicts occur that have to be solved by teamwork. This is where love really begins but this is where lust is still important.

What makes long-term romantic relationships different from our relationships with our family or friends is that special something, that physical attraction you feel to the other person. You want to be in their company and you want to get up close and personal. You might call that lust, but it is really a craving, a hunger for the other person. It includes things like holding hands, cuddling, kissing, paying attention to each other, paying compliments to each other, being attentive, being interested in your partner. So it's not just physical closeness, it's emotional closeness.

**Susie:** What about kissing?

**Dr Rosie:** Kissing can be good exercise and a slimming aid too. A peck on the cheek uses twelve muscles and burns 12.5 kilojoules, while a deep kiss uses 29 muscles. The number of kilojoules used depends on whether it's a wrestle or a marathon! There's more brain space devoted to sensation from the lips than there is for the torso of the human body. When lips meet, nerve endings zing with pleasure. Special attractors called semiochemicals secreted on the top lip are transferred when we kiss, creating bonds of attachment and love. Insurance studies have found you're less likely to be involved in a car accident on the way to work if you kiss your spouse goodbye. Wouldn't it be great if kissing lowered our insurance premiums!

**Susie:** With all those healthy reasons to have more sex, do you have some tips on how couples can get their sex life back on track?

**Dr Rosie:** Women have more muted sexual desire than men and they will often rely on other reasons to have sex apart from lust. Most women need to rely on the goodwill in the relationship to trigger interest in sexual activity. If there is no goodwill in the relationship, if he doesn't treat her nicely outside the bedroom, there won't be any sex inside the bedroom.

Often sexual problems are triggered by relationship unhappiness. A lot of people who are having problems with sex are having problems with communication, intimacy and sensuality. In other words, they're not putting enough time, energy and effort into their relationship. They're not spending enough time together, they're not talking enough, they're not emotionally close, they have drifted apart. They are not physically close, so they feel awkward together and then they wonder why sex doesn't happen.

So you have to start out with the basics if you want to have a satisfying sex life. I'm not talking about hearts and flowers and all the rest of it, I'm just talking about everyday conversation, treating each other with respect, being polite and considerate.

**Susie:** What can a man do specifically?

**Dr Rosie:** Spend time talking and listening and don't only do it when you want more sex – she'll soon wise up! Women need emotional closeness every day.

Stop hassling for sex. Nagging is NOT an aphrodisiac!

Remember grooming is even more important in the bedroom. No woman wants to go to bed with a dishevelled or smelly man.

Reassure her. Jealousy and insecurity will inhibit a woman's sex drive.

Work hard to build trust in your relationship by telling the truth and being there for her. Accept that you might always be the sexual initiator.

Make sex more enticing for her. Find out exactly what she prefers in bed.

**Susie:** What are some of your tips for women?

**Dr Rosie:** Be sensitive when he approaches you for sex. Don't reject him abruptly. Men are very vulnerable when they are sexually needy. Instead of automatically saying no to sex, contemplate the idea of having some sort of sexual activity, even if it's only manual stimulation. Sex doesn't always have to be intercourse.

Accept that your libido is likely to remain lower than his. Even if you're never overcome with 'flames of sexual desire' there are many good reasons, as we've already discussed, to engage in sex including feeling closer to your partner emotionally, expressing your love and affection, not to forget relaxing and having fun.

Make sex a higher priority in your life by leaving some time and energy for it in your daily schedule. Seek medical advice if you are experiencing menopausal dryness and any discomfort during intercourse. Lubricant will help and hormonal vaginal pessaries may be necessary.

Raise his thrill-o-meter. Be a tease. Build sexual tension by flashing him some flesh or make a sexy phone call to him at work. Tell him what you're going to do to him later that night and he'll simmer.

While a slow build-up to orgasm can be fabulous, there are few men who don't enjoy a quickie. It's all about animal instinct and unbridled passion. His levels of testosterone peak first thing in the morning. One weekend morning when he's most relaxed take him by surprise and initiate sex.

Get a grip. When he's inside you, heighten his pleasure by contracting your pelvic floor muscles around his penis. If your muscles aren't in good shape, now's the time to start a pelvic floor exercise program. The great news is these exercises increase the strength of your orgasms too.

**Susie:** Are there any true aphrodisiacs?

**Dr Rosie:** There are more than 900 supposed desire arousers recorded. That is certainly a testament to human gullibility! However, I believe that love, pure deep love is the only one true aphrodisiac. Isn't that the name of a song?

**Susie:** Carrying extra weight can have a damaging effect on our sexual self-esteem, any tips on how we can start feeling sexy about ourselves again, regardless of our shape and size?

**Dr Rosie:** So you don't have breasts like Pamela Anderson, legs like Elle Macpherson or Kylie's bum. Join the club! Research suggests that two thirds of women today are dissatisfied with their weight. The good news is that you don't have to be beautiful or have a perfect body to be sexually attractive to men. Men are first attracted to a woman's face, smile and eyes ahead of her breasts, legs and bottom. In fact, according to experts, most men are uneasy and shy around overly beautiful women.

Poor body image impairs sexual functioning in women by reducing their sexual desire and inhibiting their sexual enjoyment. A woman who is worried about how she looks when she's making love is turning herself off rather than on and will have fewer orgasms.

In the past, larger women were usually considered to be attractive, voluptuous and seductive. It's only recently that this obsession with thinness has taken over. No doubt sometime in the future, larger women will be in vogue once again. Don't be a victim of society's fickle and ever-changing tastes. Be ahead of your time and value yourself today. You might have your dad's big arms or mum's big nose. However, those arms embrace your lover and that nose inhales his scent. Focus on how well your body functions, rather than its look.

Stop criticising yourself. Your body hears everything you think and say about it. How many times a day do you tell yourself? 'I'm too fat', or 'I'm disgusting'? When you catch yourself badmouthing your body, change your tune.

**Susie:** Can the human male really be monogamous?

**Dr Rosie:** The temptation to stray for both men and women is always there. These days more women are being unfaithful than in previous decades – what's good for the gander is obviously good enough for the goose. We all like to be desired and admired and to flirt because it's an affirmation of our desirability – the fact that we are still attractive to other people. So I don't think it's solely the province of the male. Can the human male really be monogamous? The answer is he can be if he makes up his mind to be and that's a matter of commitment. Commitment is like pregnancy – you can't be a little bit pregnant and you can't be somewhat committed. If you've had affairs in the past, you may have learnt your lesson and decided to follow the 'straight and narrow' path of fidelity. But if you've developed a taste for the excitement of affairs, you'll have a hard time giving up your cheating habits.

Infidelity can be an attempt to solve a problem: feeling a bit bored, miserable, marriage rocky, craving affection and conversation, escape from unhappiness or just some hot steamy sex … oh, if only it was so simple!

**Susie:** How many kilojoules are there in semen? Is there any way of improving the taste?

**Dr Rosie:** A single ejaculation of around 5 to 10 millilitres contains 100 to 150 kilojoules. The taste of semen varies from man to man and depends to some extent on his diet. Some women swear by a mouthful of crème de menthe or a few peppermints beforehand. This not only drowns out any taste but heightens sensation for the guy. It's worth a try.

**Susie:** What is the most sensitive part of the man's penis?

**Dr Rosie:** The most erotically sensitive part of the penis is the frenulum. That's the small vertical band of tissue on the underside of the penis between the head (glans) of the penis and the shaft. While the shaft is less sensitive than the tip, it's still a huge favourite with guys. Don't forget his nipples and scrotum. Remember, every part of his penis enjoys contact with every part of your body, so be creative!

**Susie:** Is it true that if a man is overweight or obese his penis can look smaller?

**Dr Rosie:** Yes – the penis is tethered by a ligament to the pubic bone. When a man puts on weight, fat increases in the pubic area and the penis 'sinks' into the fat and looks smaller.

**Susie:** Does the size of a man's feet, hands or nose indicate the size of his erection?

**Dr Rosie:** A study published last year in a medical journal reported that there was a correlation between the length of a man's index finger and the length of his 'maximally stretched limp penis' (which is not a pretty thought!). However, checking out his 'pointing finger', won't tell you much about what to expect in the boudoir because some penises extend dramatically during arousal while others don't change a great deal. Some versions double in length. Anyway as they say, it's not the size of the boat that counts; it's the commotion of the ocean!

**Susie:** What's Dr Rosie's recipe for a happy sex life?
**Dr Rosie:**

- Start each day with a hug
- Say 'I love you' every time you speak on the phone
- Have a weekly special date together
- Accept each other's friends and family
- Kiss unexpectedly
- Apologise sincerely
- Be forgiving
- Create rituals
- Celebrate special occasions
- Compliment freely and fully
- Drink toasts of love and commitment
- Laugh at each other's jokes
- Express affection in public
- Give with no strings attached
- Never go to bed angry
- Sleep close together
- Remember marriage is the number one cause of divorce, so make it a courtship that never ends.

# Interview with Dr Gary Aaron

**Susie:** Losing our libido is one of the unfortunate symptoms of menopause. Are there any natural things we can do to restore it?

**Dr Gary Aaron:** Libido can be a factor of your hormone levels (testosterone, DHEA, oestrogen) or it may be a psychological factor – depression, distance from your partner, erectile dysfunction in men.

   If it is a factor of hormone deficiency, supplementation of this deficiency may be sufficient to improve your libido. The most effective hormone that will improve libido is testosterone. This can be applied either as an injection periodically or as a cream to the skin, or more effectively, directly to the clitoris.

   From a psychological perspective, often what is missing in a relationship is a closeness brought about by poor communication or disagreements, causing disharmony.

**Susie:** Can any foods enhance the libido?

**Dr Gary Aaron:** Although there are a number of foods listed as aphrodisiacs, I am not aware to what degree they are successful. Examples include: oysters, chili peppers, avocado, chocolate, bananas and honey.

**Susie:** Do any foods diminish the libido?

**Dr Gary Aaron:** Once again, I am not aware that these foods truly do diminish one's libido; however the following foods are thought to affect it: diet soda, popcorn, prawns, marijuana, alcohol (especially beer), cheese and sugar.

**Susie:** What food and lifestyle changes can men make to improve their libido and performance in the bedroom?

**Dr Gary Aaron:** The following foods are thought to improve a man's libido by impacting on one or more nutritional constituent:

- Sunflower seeds and pumpkin seeds promote zinc levels which are good for boosting testosterone levels
- Maca is thought to be an aphrodisiac and being rich in B vitamins helps with energy and reduces stress

- Raw nuts like almonds and cashews are rich in the amino acid L-arginine – helping to improve the production of sex hormones
- Celery is thought to increase the level of androsterone, a naturally produced pheromone
- Meat is rich in L-Carnitine – an amino acid that can boost libido

Major lifestyle changes can also improve a man's libido and performance in the bedroom:

- Create a good self-image by losing weight and eating a healthy diet
- Exercise regularly to help with blood flow through the body
- Manage stress better – overwork and over-commitment translates into a lousy sex life.

# Sex tips from celebrity lips

Here are some fun comments and observations about sex from my celebrity contributors.

**Susie:** Do you link together sex with love, rather than sex for sex's sake?

**John Maclean:** I clearly see a huge difference just between having sex and making love. Being with someone just for the sake of having sex, I would much prefer at this point in time not to bother at all. I'm just not in the slightest bit interested.

**Susie:** People often say that they find their sex life improves when they lose weight. Is that your experience?

**Dave Gorr:** An interesting thing that I've found is that the less bulk you're carrying the more sex you can have. You feel like having sex more, I find.

**Phebe Irwin:** Me too, shame there's not someone else in the room!

**Dave Gorr:** And when you feel like having sex more, circumstances will make it work for you because you're feeling better about yourself and you're carrying less weight.

**Phebe Irwin:** And you know guys' dicks grow when they lose weight. This is true. What happens is that your stomach creeps forward and you lose length from the back, so their dick doesn't actually get any longer but because your stomach comes forward it does seem to get shorter because your stomach encroaches over the back part of your penis. There's actually a scale, ten pounds is about an inch or something like that you'll have to do your own maths. [giggles]

**Susie:** If people didn't have time to exercise, would you say have sex instead?

**Jeff Fenech:** We've always got time to have sex. You need to with your partner. There's no excuse for that. None at all. If it takes you 25 minutes to go to sleep, have sex for fifteen, trust me you'll be asleep in five minutes. So it's not a bad time!

**Wayne Pearce:** I suppose. It beats paying gym fees!

**Sandra Sully:** Absolutely. Sex is healthy. It's important on a whole range of levels. A good healthy sex life is a key ingredient to being a fulfilled human being. It does help. Why not indulge yourself in everything life has to offer? It brings a smile to the dial in so many ways.

**Trevor Hendy:** I think people should have more love and I think that'll lead to more sex. Truly, you know people should have a lot more love and understanding and patience with each other.

**Jessica Rowe:** Always!

**Fran Macpherson:** Sex is the most fantastic thing on earth. Not only does it make you feel good, it binds you together. A woman said to me once 'Tire him out before he goes to work and he's not going to look anywhere.'

**Tara Moss:** Absolutely. Well they have statistics now saying that you will be a happier person if you have sex at least once a week. It doesn't matter who you are, if you are going to have some sort of sexual communication and contact with your consenting adult partner, you will be a happier and healthier person.

**Dave Gorr:** Medical tests have shown that the more sex you have the younger you look, number one. And it's a great way to keep fit.

STILL HALF MY SIZE

Well I think that's a perfect note to finish up the final chapter and this book.

Whether you're trying to stop your Toyota Land Cruiser from turning into a Kombi van equipped with built-in annexe, or you're keen to carry less junk in your trunk, or you just want things running more smoothly under the bonnet, I hope you now feel armed with the tools you'll need to achieve and fine-tune your dream car.

While I no longer live by Mae West's mantra of 'Too much of a good thing is wonderful', I can't completely relate to Kate Moss's claim that 'Nothing tastes as good as skinny feels' either, but I think I've finally found a happy medium.

I hope this book helps you set the destination in your mind's GPS to success and you continue to steer yourself in the right direction through your life's journey. In the main, it will be a voyage that only you can take but that doesn't mean you must do it on your own. Don't be frightened to stop and ask for help or directions. It's most important to believe in yourself, be honest with yourself and keep trying. Remember life is a two-way street, so I hope you find a balance between giving and receiving. In times of self-doubt or if you ever find you are lost or you need some direction, try tuning your inner radio to W double I-FM (WII-FM) and ask yourself 'What's In It For Me?'

And now as I leave you with these final words of encouragement, it's time to take the handbrake off, and see what you can do. Good luck and always remember…

'There are no traffic jams when you go the extra mile.'
– ANON

Not 'The End'
(more like a New Beginning).

# SUGGESTED REFERENCES

Suggested tools and mind maps available for a happier and smoother life journey:

*Good Loving, Good Sex* (Arrow), Dr Rosie King

*Dangerous When Wet* (Allen & Unwin), Shelley Taylor-Smith, Ian Cockerill

*Shape Up Australia* (Harper Sports), Trevor Hendy with Samantha Riley

*Fats & Figures* (Rock Wallaby), Karen Daly

*Stop Dieting and Lose Weight* (Di Harris), Di Harris

*The New Glucose Revolution* (Hodder Headline), Jennie Brand-Miller, Kaye Foster-Powell, Stephen Colagiuri

*The glucose revolution: G.I. Plus* (Hodder Headline), Jennie Brand-Miller and Kaye Foster-Powell

*Good Girls Do Swallow* (Random House), Rachael Oakes-Ash

*Bessie's Body Secrets* (New Holland), Bessie Bardot

Weight Watchers www.weightwatchers.com.au

The CEDRIC Centre (Community Eating Disorder and Related Issues Counselling) www.cedriccentre.com

*Taming the Black Dog – A Guide to Overcoming Depression* (GSK), Bev Aisbett. www.gsk.com

*Dieting – A Dry Drunk* (BLJ Nautilus) Becky Lu Jackson

*Power Up Your People Skills* (Allen & Unwin), Doug Malouf

*Switch on Your Magnetic Personality* (Rial Publishing), Doug Malouf, www.dougspeak.com

*Simply Too Good To Be True Cookbooks* (Simply Too Good Pty Ltd), Annette Sym, www.symplytoogood.com.au

*Succeed With Me – Life's little positive thinking book* (New Holland), Selwa Anthony

*Dr Rosie King's Pelvic Floor Workout* is available through mail order from the Written Word – Resources for Health Professionals telephone 1800 636748 or online at www.intimatesolutions.com.au

Snack Break: Dairy Farmer's Yoghurt, *The Checkout*, ABC1, www.youtube.com/watch?v=HUPMAlNHBiU

*Fat for Fuel* (Hay House), Dr Joseph Mercola

*Sweet Poison: Why Sugar Makes Us Fat* (Penguin), David Gillespie

Dr Gary Fettke, nofructose.com

Dr Gary Aaron, Australian Menopause Centre, menopausecentre.com.au

Pete Evans, *The Paleo Way,* peteevans.com

Dr Maxwell Strong, neurolex.com.au

Glenn Chipperfield, Aqua Bladez, facebook.com/justaddwaterfitness

Janie Larmour, thecentreofyoga.com

Laureli Blyth, nlpworldwide.com

*Think Slim* (Allen & Unwin), Mark Stephens, thinkslim.com.au

Peter Powers, Hypnotist, peterpowers.com

Tim Thornton, Hypnotist, timthornton.com.au

Leon W Cowen, Academy of Applied Hypnosis, leonwcowen.com.au

Louise Smithers, CopyTight – Editing-Proofing-Copywriting-Graphic Design, louisepr@tpg.com.au

Jacqueline Hutton, Make-up Artist, GlindaWand.com.au

# A CREDIT TO THE SOURCES

Some of the quotations from this book were taken from the following sources:

*Just Do It* (The Business Library), compiled by Harry Mills

*Be Positive* (The Business Library), compiled by Harry Mills

*Sales Secrets* (The Business Library), compiled by Harry Mills

*Zen Soup* (Penguin), Laurence G Boldt

www.gadzillion.com

# ACKNOWLEDGMENTS

There are so many people that I will be eternally grateful to for all their help. By listing some people I run the risk of forgetting others, and my humblest apologies if I have.

Thanks hugely to Bert Newton for the fantastic foreword and to all my wonderful contributors: Dr Rosie King, Shelley Taylor-Smith, Fran Macpherson, Tara Moss, Sandra Sully, Jessica Rowe, Phebe Irwin, Belinda Rolland, Janie Larmour, Laureli Blyth, Glenn Chipperfield, Christopher Essex, John Maclean OAM, Jeff Fenech, Wayne Pearce, Trevor Hendy, Dave Gorr, Pete Evans, Dr Gary Fettke, Dr Gary Aaron, Dr Maxwell Strong.

Huge thanks also go to Fiona Schultz, Alan Whiticker, Liz Hardy, Andrew Davies and all the wonderful team at New Holland Publishers, as well as Susie Smith, Dr Jim Turner and Dr Lesley Yee, Geoff Sheehan, Amanda Logan, Jacqueline Hutton, Louise Smithers, Sue Huff and my authors' agent Selwa Anthony.

# COMPARATIVE ENERGY CONSUMPTION CHART

## Comparative energy consumption (METs)

Sexual intercourse with longstanding partner

| | |
|---|---|
| Normal | 2–3 |
| Vigorous | 5–6 |
| Orgasm | 4–5 |

| | |
|---|---|
| Light housework – sweeping, polishing, ironing | 2–4 |
| Walking one kilometre on the flat for 15 minustes | 3–4 |
| Cleaning windows | 3–4 |
| Gardening – weeding | 3–5 |
| Gardening – raking | 3–6 |
| Heavy housework – making beds, scrubbing floors | 3–6 |
| Dancing – social and square | 3–7 |
| Mowing lawn | 4–5 |
| Golf | 4–5 |
| Swimming | 4–8 |
| Cycling 16 km/hr | 6–7 |
| Touch football | 6–10 |
| Shovelling 10/minute | 10 |
| Squash | 8–10 |
| Jogging | 7–15 |

# Rule of thumb for assessing CV fitness before resuming sexual intercourse

A man is fit enough for sex if he is able to:
- walk 1km on the flat in 15 minutes and
- climb two flights of stairs (20 steps) in 10 seconds
- without chest discomfort or pain, or undue breathlessness

20 steps in 10 seconds

1km on the flat in 15 minutes

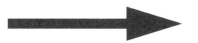

METs equivalent to intercourse     METs equivalent to orgasm

# GLENN CHIPPERFIELD'S QUICK AND EASY 'TV COMMERCIAL BREAK' EXERCISES

## Seated exercises

Be sure to breathe deeply while doing these.

- Simply get up from your seat and sit down repeatedly while holding in your core stomach muscles (bottom/thighs)
- Squats – grab knees if needed (bottom/thighs)
- Leg extension – straighten and hold leg off the ground for two counts then alternate legs (upper thighs)

## Standing exercises

- Use back of lounge to do modified push-ups (chest/arm)
- Use back of lounge to balance whilst raising up on toes (lower leg)
- Stand and lift knee up to chest (stomach)
- Hold lounge and lower self by bending knees (upper legs/ bottom)

## Standing or sitting arm exercises

(Increase intensity by holding cans or plastic bottles and increase the weight by filling them with liquid.)

- Alternate raising each arm out to the side and up to shoulder height
- Alternate raising each arm straight out in front (shoulder)
- Lean forward and alternate raising each arm back (upper back)
- Lean forward and row both arms backwards (upper back)
- Bend alternate arms up to your shoulder (biceps)

## Lying down exercises

- On your back, bend legs, feet flat on the floor, try and slide your palms up your thighs to knees (tummy)
- Bend alternate legs up to chest (lower tummy)
- Bend legs, feet flat on floor, breathe deeply as you slightly raise your bottom off the floor

To find out more about Glenn Chipperfield's Aqua Bladez and his journey in fitness follow his business Just Add Water Fitness on Facebook: facebook.com/justaddwaterfitness

Glenn's email: chipper@australiamail.com Mobile: 0418734446

# APPENDIX III

# FRAN MACPHERSON'S LOW-FAT RECIPES

## SOUPS AND STARTERS

**Fran's favourite noodle vegetable soup**
1 onion, chopped
500 ml of chicken stock (or vegetable stock, if you prefer)
Selection of vegetables cut into bite-sized pieces e.g. snow peas,
Asian greens, carrots (thinly sliced), broccoli
1 packet of fat-free noodles
1 tsp bottled chilli (optional)

Place onion in a non-stick pan, add a half teaspoon of olive oil if
desired and cook over medium heat, stirring regularly, until golden.
Turn heat up to high, add a quarter of a cup of water and cook until
water has evaporated. If using carrots, add them to the onion and
cook for a further few minutes. Add the chicken stock, bring to the
boil and allow the soup to boil for about five minutes, or until the
onion is cooked. Add the prepared vegetables and cook for about
1 minute. Soak the noodles in boiling water for 2–3 minutes before

adding them to the soup. Add the chilli and continue cooking for a just a couple more minutes, so that the vegetables stay firm. If you like you can add a little sliced, cooked chicken, beef, tofu or prawns at the end. Serves 1–2 people.

## Broccoli soup

1 large onion chopped
1 large head of broccoli, chopped into small pieces
1 very small washed new potato, chopped into cubes but not peeled
500 ml chicken stock (can be vegetable or beef stock)

Place all of the vegetables and the stock in a large saucepan over high heat and boil for about 30 minutes, or until all the vegetables are thoroughly cooked. Use a hand-held blender to blend the soup until smooth or transfer to a blender or food processor. Add freshly ground pepper and a little salt before serving. The soup should be really thick and you can replace the broccoli with pumpkin or cauliflower. Serves 2.

## Yum yum tofu

1 packet of firm tofu
½ teaspoon olive oil
Asian greens
Sweet soy sauce, to serve

Slice the tofu into ½ cm slices. Use your hands to wipe the olive oil over the firm tofu. Place the tofu on foil under a hot grill and grill on both sides until golden. In the meantime, prepare and wash the Asian greens and stir-fry in a wok or frying pan with a little oil. Add a little water, cover and steam for a minute or two. Pile greens on a plate, put the tofu on top and pour a little sweet soy sauce over the top. Serves 2.

## Asparagus with low-fat ricotta

1 bunch asparagus, ends trimmed
100 g low-fat ricotta cheese
Chilli sauce, if desired

Preheat oven to 220° C. Place asparagus in a single layer in an ovenproof serving dish. Spread low-fat ricotta over asparagus, sprinkle with chilli sauce if desired. Bake for about 5 minutes. If you prefer, you can place the dish under a grill for about 8 minutes. Serves 2.

## Ratatouille

4 tomatoes, chopped
2 onions (one red and one brown), chopped
1 medium eggplant, chopped
2 zucchini, sliced
1 red or green capsicum, chopped
1 medium red chilli, finely chopped

Make sure that all of the vegetables other than the onion are about the same size. Preheat oven to about 170° C. Mix vegetables together in an oven bag, add ground pepper and a little salt. Tie the oven bag and pierce a couple of times near the tie. Place bag in a baking dish and cook for about 1 hour. Serves 4 as a side dish.

## Stuffed capsicum

2 large red or green capsicum
Ratatouille mix, as before, uncooked
Handful of shiitake or Swiss brown mushrooms, sliced

Preheat oven to around 180° C. Halve capsicums horizontally and remove seeds. Stuff with ratatouille mix. Top with mushrooms and sprinkle with a little olive oil, and freshly ground pepper and sea salt. Place in a baking dish on baking paper and cook for around 45 minutes. You can also stuff large mushrooms. Don't wash the mushrooms, chop the stalk and add to ratatouille mix, stuff as for capsicums and top with sliced pitted olives.

## Sunday eggs with ratatouille

Put previously cooked ratatouille in a two-cup ramekin. Break one or two eggs over the top. Top with plastic, place in microwave and cook for a couple of minutes on high. Alternatively, cover with foil and cook in a medium oven for about 10 minutes.

**Raw salmon heaven**

1 salmon fillet, skin and bones removed

2 small red chillies, finely chopped

2 stalks of celery, finely chopped

½ red capsicum, diced

1 red onion, finely chopped 1 tbsp capers

Juice of 1 lemon and 1 lime (if available)

Combine vegetables with lemon and lime juice. Place fish in a shallow dish and top with vegetable mix. Place in fridge for at least 30 minutes. Serve with crackers, with green leaves for a starter or stir through fat-free noodles or spaghetti.

# MAIN MEALS

**Tuna salad**

1 tin good quality tuna in oil

1 tin cannellini beans

2 stalks celery, finely chopped

½ red capsicum, chopped

1 red onion, chopped

1 red chilli, finely chopped

1 tbsp capers

1 tbsp chilli sauce

Juice of 1 lemon

Drain tuna well, reserving oil. Place tuna in a bowl and add celery, capsicum, onion and chilli. Drain and wash cannellini beans and add to tuna mix. Add capers and chilli sauce. Mix well then add lemon juice. Pour a little of the reserved tuna oil over the salad. You can adjust the amount of lemon juice to taste.

**Lamb shanks**

1 lamb shank per person (buy the 'Frenched' shanks from the butcher, they are trimmed of all fat and gristle)

1 tin chopped tomatoes

2 fresh tomatoes, chopped

1 brown onion, chopped or two small pickling onions per person,
left whole 2 cloves of garlic, chopped
½ cup red wine
250 ml beef stock
1 tbsp plain flour.

Preheat oven to around 170° C. Place flour in a large oven bag, add
lamb shanks, and shake until coated. Add all other ingredients. Tie
up top of bag and pierce a couple of times near tie. Place bag in
a baking dish or on a baking tray and bake for around 90 minutes.
Serve with broccolini and beans and green herbs mixed with a little
grainy mustard and cooked in the microwave on high for about three
minutes.

**Baked fish**
1 salmon or trout fillet per person or 1 whole baby trout
2 green onions
2cm piece of ginger, sliced
1 lemon, thinly sliced
1 lemon for juice

Preheat oven to 180° C. Put each fillet on foil that is big enough to
make a parcel. Cover the fish with green onions, then cover these
with ginger slices. Squeeze lemon juice over fish and, finally, top with
lemon slices. Roll up foil into parcels, place parcels on a baking tray
and bake for about 10 minutes or until cooked through. If using
whole trout, bake for about 20 minutes. Serve with wilted Chinese
greens cooked in non-stick wok in a little water with the lid tightly
on. Add a little soy sauce to the greens at end of cooking.

# DESSERT

**Medley of mixed fruit with yoghurt**
1 packet mixed dried fruit, sliced or chopped
1 cup water or fruit juice (apple is best)
250 g tub of good quality low-fat yoghurt
Preheat oven to 170° C. Combine water or fruit juice with dried fruit

mix and place in an oven bag. Tie up bag and pierce a couple of times near the tie. Place bag in a baking dish or baking tray and bake for about 45 minutes. Meanwhile, beat yoghurt with an eggbeater or Mixmaster. Place in a bowl and freeze until firm. Serve with the fruit mix, as you would ice cream. You can also add strawberry or other fruit puree if desired.

### Baked pears

1 large pear per person, halved and cored
½ cup golden syrup
1 tsp grated ginger

Preheat oven to 200° C. Mix golden syrup with grated ginger and drizzle over pears. Place pears on a baking tray lined with baking paper and bake for about 45 minutes. Serve with yoghurt.

# ABOUT THE AUTHOR

Susie Elelman is truly the epitome of a multimedia broadcaster and has been deservedly described as the most versatile, informed and professional person in Australian media today. Author, TV presenter, radio broadcaster, reporter and producer are just some of the many hats she has worn throughout an impressive media career spanning four decades.

Susie Elelman is a name synonymous with daytime television and can currently be seen voicing her opinions as a regular co-host on *Studio 10*.

Susie's long list of television credits include more than eight years spent alongside Bert Newton as a presenter and reporter on *Good Morning Australia* and seven years with Larry Emdur and Kylie Gillies on *The Morning Show*.

Susie was host and executive producer of her own national, daily, variety and lifestyle show *SUSIE* and then co-hosted and co-produced the national live news and current affairs show *DAILY* with Susie and Bianca both on the WIN/9 network. Susie also went head to head with Stan Zemanek as a long-standing panellist on Network 10 and Foxtel's *Beauty and the Beast*.

Susie's television career has seen her chat one-to-one with many international stars and she counts Tom Cruise, Nicole Kidman, Whoopi Goldberg, Audrey Hepburn, Kylie Minogue and George Clooney among the celebrities she has interviewed.

An established presence on national radio, Susie regularly formed part of the 2GB talkback team on Sydney's number one radio station and 4BC Brisbane along with various stations on the Macquarie Network.

Without touching that remote control Susie can move her skills to be your emcee or corporate communicator and business educator. Bringing her signature charm and effervescent enthusiasm to every event, Susie can always be relied upon to deliver a powerful message with panache.

For her services to charity, the not-for-profit sector and the media Susie was extremely humbled and honoured to be awarded an AM (Member of the Order of Australia Medal) in the Queen's Birthday honours list in June 2015.

*Still Half My Size* is Susie's second book.